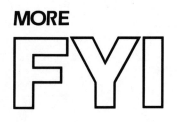

MORE

MORE

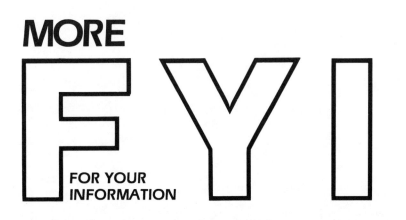

F Y I

**FOR YOUR
INFORMATION**

Further Tips for Healthful Living

based on the award-winning ABC-TV program

with HAL LINDEN

EDITED BY NAT BRANDT
WRITTEN BY
    Alton Blakeslee
    Tabitha Powledge
    Judith N. Schwartz
    Linda Sutter

M. EVANS AND COMPANY, INC., New York

Library of Congress Cataloging in Publication Data
Main entry under title:

More FYI.

Continues: FYI.
Includes index.
1. Health—Miscellanea. I. Linden, Hal.
II. Brandt, Nat. III. Blakeslee, Alton L. IV. FYI
(Television program) V. FYI.
RA776.M85   1983   613   83-14171

ISBN 0-87131-424-X
ISBN 0-87131-420-7 (pbk.)

M. Evans and Company, Inc.
216 East 49 Street
New York, New York 10017

Design by Ronald F. Shey

Manufactured in the United States of America

Foreword by Hal Linden

It's not the eyes that go first. Or the legs. It's the . . . er . . . the er . . . oh yes . . . the memory!

I don't know how memory operates as a brain function (I'm not too sure anyone does), but I've discovered that I remember things from twenty-five years ago—facts, names, places, faces— a lot more distinctly than from, say, five to ten years ago. Now, that may seem illogical. One would imagine recency would help. But although I can remember the names of the cast of *Bells Are Ringing* (my first Broadway show) down to the assistant stage managers, I have difficulty recalling almost anyone from my last Broadway show (a revival of *The Pajama Game*) other than the producer, the director, and my co-stars.

I'm sure there are those who would offer psychological explanations for this phenomenon, but I've come up with my own theory. I look upon my brain as a blackboard on which impressions are chalked. When the blackboard was relatively clean, the words could be written neatly and read easily. As time progressed and impressions multiplied, it became more difficult to find open space, and the words were either compressed or overlapped other words. By now it's practically white-on-white, and it's tough to read anything.

To deal with this problem, I have developed a technique I call "creative forgetting." It involves selectively erasing words from the blackboard (neatly, no smudges; that only makes things worse) and introducing new words—but instead of in chalk, in a sort of disappearing ink, which remains legible as long as I need it and then discreetly goes away. I used this technique quite successfully while taping *Barney Miller*. We made, after all, 170 episodes. Each week I memorized my lines quickly, and generally accurately. But on the following Monday, as we read the new script, I was able to clear my head (blackboard) and start all over. Not only could I not recall any lines from last week's show, I was hard pressed to remember what the show was about.

All of the foregoing is by way of explaining why, when I open a letter from a viewer that reads: "On Tuesday, on Channel 3, you said something about arthritis and sex. I'm sixty-seven and my wife . . . ," it's not that I'm dispassionate about geriatric passion (on the contrary, I look forward to it eagerly, especially as the future becomes decidedly more and more not-too-distant), it's just that I can't be of help. I remember talking about arthritis and sex, but the details were delibly written on my blackboard in disappearing ink. And by necessity. We have, to this date, created six hundred *FYI* spots. Can you imagine the mess if I had used chalk on the blackboard? Not to mention the dust!

But rest assured, my loyal Channel 3 viewer, your letter was not ignored. It went back to the same excellent research staff who amassed the material that led to the original spot, and it was from that staff you received an informed response.

To those of you who don't feel like writing and/or waiting for the information, I recommend the same information source that I now keep readily at hand—this book!

HAL LINDEN
Los Angeles

Preface

FYI, ABC's award-winning series, is now in its fourth year. The mini-programs (each is forty-five seconds long) receive five hundred to a thousand letters each week from viewers asking for information, using *FYI* as a resource. And occasionally there is a touching and moving letter, telling, for example, how *FYI* saved one woman from unnecessary surgery, how it prompted another to take her child to the dentist to save a tooth, how it cured a boy of bedwetting and a man of migraines. It has been a heartening response. And as we suspected, the first book served not only the show's television audience but also thousands of other people who had never seen *FYI* but found its serendipitous collection of information helpful.

At the foundation of *FYI* is its research staff and consultants. Three researchers and thirteen consultants are constantly looking for material, checking, rechecking, and triple-checking everything we report. In the last four years *FYI* has amassed an enormous file of material—important material. Clearly, we cannot possibly produce enough mini-programs to keep up with this volume of information. *More FYI* is an attempt to let the reader benefit from all this research. As a result, this book is a mixture of information based on the television show and culled from our files.

Our thanks to ABC and particularly to Jacqueline Smith, Vice President of Daytime, for her continued support and encouragement; to her associates, Jean Arley and Randi LeWinter; to Mary Ann Donahue and to the entire staff and consultants of *FYI*, listed in the back of the book, who keep the show alive and well; to Jean Barish, for her dedication to accuracy; to Joe Gustaitis, Robin Westen, and Elaine Brown Whitley for their talent in finding new and fresh material for *FYI*, and to Elinor Bunin for her support and creative dedication to *FYI*. And last but not least, our thanks to Susan Garbarini Fanning, who as the editorial assistant worked closely with the editor and kept everything running smoothly from research to final product.

NAT BRANDT, Editor
YANNA KROYT BRANDT, Producer, *FYI*
New York City

How to Use This Book

This second *FYI* book, like the television show, offers advice on healthful living. In question-and-answer form, you will find some of the latest information on subjects such as keeping fit, eating well, and staying healthy. Following the questions and answers is a section with brief updates of selected items from the first book. There are also four appendixes, which supplement certain entries. For those readers who want specific information about a particular topic, there is a detailed index at the back of the book. So whether you are reading for pleasure or are in search of the latest information about nutrition, you can find what you're looking for.

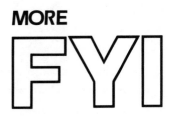

MORE

Can you relax away acne?

Quite possibly. Doctors have now found out why ointments and special diets haven't helped to cure many people's skin problems: almost 80 percent of all such problems may be emotional.

Emotion—including being tense or upset—produces changes in the body's chemistry, and no matter what ointment you use, no matter what diet you follow, your skin disorder will most likely persist. That is, unless you take a different tack and learn to relax—which you can do.

The skin is a sensitive transmitter of feelings. Your first contact with the world as an infant is through your skin. Your first response to another human being is to your mother's skin, as you're held close. As you mature and your sexuality develops, the skin's surface becomes very sensitive to many of your emotions—anger, excitement, despair, tension. In response, it blushes, blanches, prickles, sweats, gets goosebumps and rashes, merely from a normal range of events. Undue or abnormal tension can erupt into acne.

There are two ways in which you can help yourself: exercise and relaxation. Many doctors believe exercise is important because it suffuses the skin with blood, which provides more nutrients, releases sweat, and increases the oxygen supply.

Regular, self-induced relaxation can also be helpful. One way to help yourself is to try deep-breathing exercises. Another is through meditation. If you need help, meditation tapes and cassettes are available; ask your dermatologist about them.

What do dry skin, falling hair, and a fast pulse have in common?

A tiny gland weighing less than an ounce. It's the thyroid gland—shaped like a butterfly and straddling the windpipe—which secretes less than $1/100,000$ ounce of the hormone thyroxine a day, yet affects virtually every system in your body.

Too much or too little hormone can set off a variety of debilitating, sometimes dangerous symptoms—which are often traced to stress, rather than the thyroid gland. Some people have been hospitalized for psychiatric treatment when their problems were actually the result of a malfunctioning thyroid. But now there are simple blood tests to detect thyroid abnormalities.

Thyroxine affects your appetite, your heart, your muscles and skin, your eyes and nervous system, your ability to sweat and to reproduce, even your personality. It also controls the rate at which cells of your body use calories—the metabolic rate. With too much hormone, the rate goes up. That may increase your appetite, but you'll end up losing weight. With too little thyroid hormone, you may gain weight.

Thyroid deficiency can bring about loss of hair, puffiness of hands and face, drowsiness, constipation, weight gain, slowed reflexes, and, in women, menstrual changes and the chance of miscarriage. In children thyroid deficiency may show up as tiredness, inability to concentrate, and, in extreme cases, stunting of growth and delay of puberty. Thyroid deficiency can be dangerous in newborns; unless it is detected and treated quickly, it can result in mental retardation and retarded growth.

Doctors now have easy and quick blood tests to measure the amount of thyroxine in the blood. They can give thyroid hormone supplements to counter a deficiency, or drugs to quiet down an overactive gland. Patients taking thyroid hormone should be tested at regular intervals to make sure their own gland hasn't recovered and is producing more hormone, along with the supplement, than they need.

So if you have an unexplained health problem, ask your doctor about new blood tests called TSH and T3, which can detect thyroid problems.

Who's finally coming into his own in the home?

Father. And high time, too. The social changes of recent years—new, less rigid attitudes about the proper roles for men and women, and the practical fact that so many mothers of young children work outside the home—have made Dad an important person.

Child psychologists, pediatricians, and other professionals are discovering what many successful families have always known: Fathers and children are good for each other. In fact, in the United

States close to a million children are now being raised by fathers alone. Even so, many men are fearful and uncertain about succeeding at becoming more involved fathers.

As would be expected, Dad still does not spend nearly as much time with the kids as Mom does. One recent study of infants between six and twelve months found that mothers averaged nine hours a day with them, while fathers were with them for only a little over three hours.

The realities of earning a living prevent many fathers from spending as much time with their children as they'd like, but they can take heart from the words of Ross D. Parke, author of *Fathers:* "The real question is not how many hours per day a father spends with his child, but what he does with the child when he *is* present." Pop can, and should, use that precious time, however brief, to encourage exploration, to introduce interesting toys and books, to point out and talk about interesting features of the environment.

The father can begin to be a more effective parent early on by providing his wife with emotional support during pregnancy and labor, and share her joy in those times, too. He can go along on visits to the pediatrician, and ask questions. He can be aware of the fact that he's a role model for his child, and that the kind of relationship he has with his wife will serve as an example of healthy—or unhealthy—maturity and marriage.

The father can also express love and affection for his child, which men don't always find easy—and which our society has not always encouraged. Hugs and kisses are definitely in order. So are carrying and rocking, not only to relieve the mother of some chores, but also to cement his own bond with his child.

A father ordinarily tends to vigorous and energetic horseplay with boys. But girls need horseplay also. Scientific evidence indicates that successful women received a great measure of attention from their fathers.

Dad can be a teacher, too, from early language training through early adulthood and even beyond. He can let his children know he values learning, and he can keep an eye on schoolwork to make sure it's done properly. He can show up not just at the school play, but at parent-teacher conferences as well, and take an active interest in his children's educational progress. If he does this, Dr. Christopher H. Hodgman, associate professor of psychiatry and pediatrics at the University of Rochester (New York) School of Medicine, points out, "The message to child and to school personnel alike is that the father supports his child's education."

A more traditional role for father is that of disciplinarian and moralist. "Fathers, at least as much as mothers, are the repository for continuing reinforcement of social values and morality," Dr. Hodgman observes. He points out, however, that many fathers confuse discipline with punishment. But studies show that support is generally more productive than punishment in reinforcing discipline. Moreover, fathers need to remember that their own behavior as role models sets the standards of proper conduct nonverbally. "Coming to a full stop at a stop sign at an empty intersection," the doctor says, "may convey more respect for the law than would a dozen lectures on the topic."

Fathers also convey sexual identities to their children, and sexual attitudes as well, often unconsciously. Talking about sex with their children makes many fathers extremely nervous, but extensive discussions aren't necessary. Fathers can give their children a good start toward healthy sexual attitudes simply by their own secure behavior, and by giving short, informative answers to any questions their children ask.

Ideally, children need both mothers *and* fathers, say Gloria Norris and Jo Ann Miller, authors of *The Working Mother's Complete Handbook.* "Not so that they can go fishing with Dad and bake cookies with Mom, but so that they can experience tenderness and strength, guidance and affection, from two people who love them. The sharing of household management and childcare will lead, we hope, not to more fathers who 'mother' but to more actively involved male and female parents."

Can hypertensives ever cut back on drugs?

Yes, they can. They can also change drugs when necessary, even sometimes eliminate them—and look forward to a longer, healthier life than ever before. The key is proper care.

A recent five-year study by the National Heart, Lung and Blood Institute of more than ten thousand men and women with hypertension showed the benefits of reduced drug therapy. It was discovered that those who were treated in special clinics where they were intensively monitored and had their drug dosages adjusted had a 17 percent lower death rate from hypertension-associated conditions—such as heart attack, stroke, and kidney failure—than a matched group that was not followed up as intensively. Moreover, there was a 28.6 percent reduction in the death rate among those in the intensive-care group with borderline or mild hypertension.

When a drug is prescribed, it does not mean that a patient is locked into an irreversible, lifetime pattern. Dr. Frank A. Finnerty, Jr., of the George Washington University Medical School in Washington, D.C., reports that, in some cases, once blood pressure is brought down under stable control, it is often possible to lower dosages or to stop some drugs entirely, at least for a while. Besides, Dr. Finnerty found, just knowing that if you stick to your doctor's advice, take your medication, and eat properly there's a good chance you can lower your blood pressure and stop taking drugs is incentive enough for most people to stick to a strict regimen. And that can have a profound impact, because many hypertensives stop paying close attention to their doctor's advice once they begin feeling better.

Treating hypertension is largely a matter of common-sense living habits, which include maintaining good weight, exercising properly, and sticking to a low-salt or salt-free diet. As to the last, the trick is to know where salt is buried. Many prepared and processed foods are very high in sodium. Avoid them. When you need seasoning, try garlic or lemon instead. Fresh fruits and vegetables are tasty, healthy—and salt-free—foods.

When these measures are not sufficient, it may be necessary to take blood-pressure pills. There are a number of such medications and they act in different ways, so it is important to let your doctor know if the one prescribed causes you any side effects, such as memory loss, verbal impairment, depression, asthma, or, in men, impotency.

One work of caution: Don't smoke and drink caffeinated beverages when on a drug for high blood pressure. A new report from England, based on a study of mildly hypertensive caffeine drinkers who smoked between ten and thirty-five cigarettes daily, found that smoking while drinking caffeinated beverages raises blood pressure and blocks the action of medications. Curtailing both can't but help, anyway.

How can a deaf person hear?

By using one of two new devices that offer lifesaving emergency help to many deaf or hearing-impaired people.

The first is called a Tactile Communicator, and even for a person who is completely deaf, it makes hearing of a sort possible. Developed by the Helen Keller National Center for Deaf, Blind Youths and Adults, the device costs about $300 and works on the same principle as a citizen's band radio. It's made up of a small receiver, which can be worn or carried, and a transmitter the size of a clock radio, with five channels that can be tuned to five different sounds in the house, including fire alarms, doorbells, telephones, and alarm clocks. Each sound is transmitted to the receiver in coded vibrations, and each channel has a different code. The signal can be received anywhere inside or outside the house within 300 feet of the transmitter.

For example, let's say a deaf person wearing it is gardening outside the house when a burglar alarm inside rings on channel 1. Channel 1 coded vibrations are transmitted to the communicator receiver, and the person is alerted to go for help. If at the same time a home fire alarm hooked up to channel 3 should go off, it can override the other four channels, which makes it useful for an emergency signal.

The Tactile Communicator has limitations (it doesn't work with most battery-operated smoke detectors), so for further information, write to Gert Queen, Librarian, Helen Keller National Center, 111 Middle Neck Road, Sands Point, NY 11050.

The second hearing device is designed to help the estimated twenty thousand Americans who are ultra-audiometric, which means they hear only at very high frequencies. They can hear dog whistles, slamming doors, telephones, and other such sounds, but they can't hear musical notes or similar sounds, and they rely heavily on lip reading. For ultra-audiometrics, regular hearing aids are no help. If they use them, they might lose the hearing they have through overstimulation or acoustic trauma. Most of them were born with full hearing but lost their lower register because of a fever, meningitis, or other childhood disease. For many of them the problem has never been diagnosed because testing heretofore has been inadequate.

Charles I. Berlin, an audiologist who is head of the Kresge

Hearing Research Laboratory of the South in New Orleans, has developed a battery-operated miniature magnetic earphone with two channels. One channel amplifies high-pitched sounds; the other pushes lower pitches up into the ultra-audiometric range, thereby considerably enhancing a patient's ability to hear normally. If you think this device might help, you can find out more by calling a collect hotline: (301) 897-8682. When you call, ask about testing, too. Eight free ultra-audiometric testing centers have been set up throughout the country, and there is testing in a number of schools for the deaf, too.

What can pelvic pain be a sign of?

An ectopic pregnancy, if you're of childbearing age and have had intercourse. But there are now tests that can spot it early, before serious problems develop.

In a normal pregnancy, egg and sperm fuse in one of a woman's pair of fallopian tubes, the narrow channels connecting the ovaries to the uterus. The fertilized egg then migrates into the womb, where it nestles into the wall of tissue and develops into a fetus. In an ectopic pregnancy, the process goes a bit haywire. The fertilized egg embeds itself outside the uterus, most commonly in the fallopian tube, becoming a tubal pregnancy.

Such pregnancies can be catastrophic. Some women are rendered sterile by ectopic pregnancies. Tubal pregnancies can rupture, leading to hemorrhage and death; they account for more than 10 percent of maternal deaths in the United States each year, and are the chief cause of death in the first three months of pregnancy. The number of ectopic pregnancies has more than doubled in recent years, from 17,900 in 1970 to 41,000 in 1977, and they are now thought to occur in one out of every two hundred pregnancies.

Doctors suspect a number of causes for the increase. Pelvic inflammatory disease is on the rise, a result of both gonorrhea and nonvenereal infections; it can lead to scarring and eventual blockage of the fallopian tubes. The use of intrauterine devices (IUDs) to prevent pregnancy is associated with a high risk of pelvic inflammatory disease and may contribute to the incidence of ectopic pregnancy. Other factors include congenital malformations of the fallopian tubes, surgery in the abdomen–pelvic region, and perhaps the use of oral contraceptives.

The key to successful treatment is early detection so that surgery can end the pregnancy. But the symptoms can mimic those of other disorders, making diagnosis difficult. The classic warning sign is abdominal pain, sometimes accompanied by spotty vaginal bleeding or evidence of early pregnancy such as a missed menstrual period, breast changes, nausea, and frequent urination. Consult your doctor immediately if you suspect you may have an ectopic pregnancy. Diagnosis can be made early by the use of blood pregnancy tests, sonography, and laparoscopy prior to rupture of the fallopian tube.

What's the new age limit at a day-care center?

Try seventy or eighty years old. Day-care centers are not just for kids anymore.

Day care for the elderly has been described as an idea whose time has come. From a handful a decade ago, there are now more than eight hundred such centers across the country, and the number is growing. Unlike conventional senior centers, which primarily cater to the able-bodied, these centers provide such services as medical or nursing care, physical therapy, facilities for the handicapped, nutritional meals, and transportation, as well as social and recreational programs. Some of them—frequently those run by nursing homes—also offer the option of occasional overnight care. This concept, called "respite care," makes it possible for families to leave their homes without worrying about a grandparent's well-being.

Many communities now also have a range of at-home services, from nursing care to Meals on Wheels to youth volunteers who will do chores and run errands. There are organizations that help older people find roommates or even surrogate families eager to provide living space and company in exchange for help with the rent.

Most of these services are moderately priced or are covered, in full or in part, by health insurance plans. Some are free.

Information can be obtained from senior centers, hospitals,

state offices of the aging, or community or religious social service agencies.

For further information, contact:

American Health Care Association
1050 17th Street NW
Washington, DC 20005

National Association of Home Health Agencies
205 C Street NE
Washington, DC 20002

National Council on the Aging
600 Maryland Avenue SW
West Wing 100
Washington, DC 20024

Local office of the Social Security Administration
(check your phone book under "United States Government Offices")

Family Service Association of America
44 East 23rd Street
New York, NY 10010

National Association of Home Health Agencies
426 C Street NE
Washington, DC 20002

National Council for Homemaker–Home Health Aide Services, Inc.
67 Irving Place
New York, NY 10003

American Association of Homes for the Aging
Suite 770
1050 17th Street NW
Washington, DC 20036

American Association of Retired Persons
1909 K Street NW
Washington, DC 20049

Gray Panthers
3635 Chestnut Street
Philadelphia, PA 19104

What's the ringer in exercise for the elderly?

Horseshoes. According to Dr. Sol Berman, an orthopedic surgeon from New Jersey and a nine-time horseshoe champion of his state who is in his seventies, horseshoe pitching is an ideal sport for older people. It promotes fat metabolism more efficiently than jogging, helping to lower cholesterol levels and fight hardening of the arteries. It strengthens the hands, wrists, arms, shoulders, back, and legs, and helps maintain healthy bones.

Pitching horseshoes is also excellent rehabilitation for those who have had heart attacks—and good for pregnant women and the handicapped, too, because how long and hard it's played is up to the players. And because horseshoes are light, only two and a half pounds, there's little chance of strain.

As one gets better one can play harder and longer. A good, rousing game will involve more walking than golf and more bending than tennis doubles. If you get to play in a tournament, as Dr. Berman does, you might, he calculates, walk five miles, bend five hundred times, and throw more than a ton of steel—and enjoy it.

Horseshoes are cheap. All you need is a backyard or a fair-sized garage to play in. So try for a ringer around the horseshoe stake. It's good for health, for morale—and for three points.

What's poisonous about a philodendron and some other plants?

Just about everything. According to medical specialists, the leaves, stems, flowers, roots, and other parts of more than seven hundred different kinds of plants that grow in the United States contain toxic substances that can prove deadly if ingested.

The plants pose a particular danger to children, who have a tendency to put objects in their mouth. In fact, after medicines, plants are the leading cause of poisoning among children under five years old.

Poisonous plants do not have to grow wild or be exotic; many are familiar favorites found in homes and gardens. Among them:

18

philodendron, English ivy, dieffenbachia, sweet pea, morning glory, azalea, hyacinth, daffodil, iris, hydrangea, and rhododendron. (For a list of toxic parts and symptoms associated with fifty common plants, see Appendix C.)

When eaten, poisonous plants can produce ill effects ranging from swelling of the tongue and lips, nausea, vomiting, and diarrhea to cramps, convulsions, and even heartbeat irregularities. The poisons are sometimes so potent that even a tiny taste can be deadly. For example, a single leaf of the oleander plant contains enough of a chemical active on heart tissue to kill an adult. Using a branch of the plant as a barbecue stick can deposit enough of the substance on meat to kill a child.

Doctors offer parents several suggestions to safeguard their youngsters' health:

☐ Know the names of the plants you have and label the containers they grow in.

☐ Keep household plants out of a child's reach.

☐ Warn your youngsters against eating plants or playing with them—for example, using hollow stems to make peashooters or whistles.

☐ Post the number of the nearest poison control center by the telephone and call it immediately if you suspect your child has eaten a harmful plant. The medically trained staff will tell you what to do.

Can you eat the blues away?

You can certainly help to chase them with the proper diet.

Like every other part of our bodies, our brains are made of substances that come from the foods we eat. Common sense dictates that what we eat will affect all our functions, including our moods. But it is only in the last decade or so that scientists have begun to gain insight into what the brain chemicals are, how they work, and how nutrition influences their activity.

One important brain chemical is the neurotransmitter serotonin, which sends messages along the nerve pathways. Too low a level of serotonin has been correlated with, among other disorders, depression and sleeplessness, although it is not the only factor in those conditions. The body makes serotonin from tryptophan, an amino acid or subunit of protein, which we get from protein-rich foods.

Among the tryptophan foods that nutrition experts think may help relieve mild depression (and possibly premenstrual tension) are turkey, chicken, bananas, cheese, pineapple, and yogurt. They should be combined with foods high in the stress-fighting B vitamins, such as whole grains, green leafy vegetables, organ meats, and brown rice. Carbohydrate foods like pasta work too, because they increase the body's output of insulin, which allows the small amount of tryptophan in the food to get to the brain and be converted to serotonin.

When your spirits are low, it may be wise to avoid foods such as lobster, egg yolks, and marbled meats, which contain choline, a chemical that can be a downer.

Too much sugar and salt also affect mood: sugar because in excess it can cause overproduction of insulin, salt because it can lead to excessive water retention.

Be sure your daily diet includes all the essential nutrients—vitamins, minerals, protein, carbohydrates, and whole-grain and dairy products. Balance proteins and carbohydrates, and avoid choline-rich foods. As Dr. Brian L. G. Morgan, an assistant professor of nutrition at Columbia University, says: "By manipulating diet, changing the amount of carbohydrate or protein you eat just a little, you can have quite a profound and dramatic effect on how you feel."

Is a second heart attack inevitable?

Not anymore. Two new classes of drugs promise to increase dramatically the chances of survival for hundreds of thousands of heart-attack patients. Some 350,000 Americans survive a first heart attack each year, but one in seven dies of a second attack within two years. The new drugs are expected to revise those grim statistics.

Of the 350,000, the National Institutes of Health estimates that 230,000 or more can be treated with beta-adrenergic blockers, a class of drugs that lower the heart's workload and drop blood pressure by blocking the effect of adrenaline and other heart-stimulating chemicals. Six beta blockers are available for use in the United States: propranolol (trade name Inderal), metoprolol (Lopressor), nadolol (Corgard), atenolol (Tenormin), timolol (Blocadren), and pindolol (Visken). Others are being used extensively abroad and will likely be approved here later.

The six now available have been used for years in Europe, but conservative American drug policies delayed their use here until the first was approved in 1981. Death rates dropped 26 percent in an American study of propranolol by the National Heart, Lung and Blood Institute. Tests with other beta blockers reduced deaths by 36 percent in Sweden and 39 percent in Norway.

The second class of new drugs is called calcium-entry blockers. They block calcium ions (charged atoms) that make heart-muscle tissue constrict, thereby increasing the flow of blood to heart muscle. Three of these approved for use in this country are verapamil (Isoptin), nifedipine (Procardia), and diltiazem hydrochloride (Cardiazem).

The calcium-entry blockers are not intended to replace existing methods of treatment, but rather to augment and to supplement therapy with such agents as the beta-adrenergic blockers. Some doctors have found that the combination works better than either type of drug used alone.

One note of caution: A team of British doctors, after studying the effects of a beta blocker called oxprenolol, warn that the use of beta blockers increases the chances of coronary death in a man if treatment is delayed for more than a year after the man has been stricken. Their conclusion—published in the *New England Journal of Medicine* and based on a study of more than 1,100 males between thirty-five and sixty-nine years old who survived heart attacks—is that to be effective, treatment should be started within a few weeks after a first attack.

Can babies be treated before birth?

Yes. Within the last decade doctors have crossed a brave new frontier and begun treating fetuses in the womb. Though this fetal therapy is still in the experimental stage and has met so far with mixed success, it offers great hope of an alternative to two harrowing options once an abnormality has been diagnosed: an abortion or the birth of a child with physical and/or mental defects.

Since the 1960s doctors have been giving blood transfusions into the abdomen of the fetus to treat Rh blood incompatibility between mother and fetus. More recently they have begun to infuse endangered fetuses with vitamins and drugs as well. For example, at the University of California in San Francisco a fetus unable to properly use the vitamin biotin was treated successfully by giving the mother-to-be massive injections of the vitamin daily for the last three months of her pregnancy.

More spectacularly, a variety of drugs can be injected directly into the amniotic sac that cushions the fetus, which absorbs the medications, among them digitalis for abnormal heart rhythms, a thyroid hormone for thyroid deficiency, and a drug to help lungs mature so that the baby will not have difficulty breathing when a premature birth is likely.

The most dramatic development has occurred within the last few years as doctors have begun to operate on the fetus in the womb. Only a handful of centers are doing such work, most prominently the University of Colorado and the Medical College of Virginia. Fewer than fifty tiny patients have been treated. So far the operations have been limited in scope—either momentary insertions of needles or the implantation of tubes into the fetus to drain excess fluid from such areas as the kidneys, bladder, chest, abdomen, lungs, and even the brain. The tubes are removed after birth.

The pressure of fluid buildup can cause physical deformities and mental defects and lead to a child's early death. Recently physicians took a more ambitious step, performing an out-of-womb operation on a fetus with an obstructed urinary tract. The doctors removed the fetus from the uterus, operated, and returned it to the womb. Though the pregnancy continued to term, the baby died soon after birth because the condition had progressed too far for the surgery to correct it.

What makes fetal therapy possible is the availability of sophisticated prenatal diagnostic techniques, including ultrasound and amniocentesis, and, in the case of fetal surgery, the development of a new and powerful drug, ritodrine, that prevents a woman from going into premature labor. In the future, doctors hope, they will be able to transplant into the fetus entire organs or tissues that can stimulate bone growth or manufacture missing essential chemicals. But for now that is a long time off.

There are now eight treatment centers in the United States that perform fetal surgery:

Division of Maternal and Fetal Medicine
Georgetown University
Washington, DC 20057

Department of Pediatric Surgery
University of California
San Francisco, CA 94143

Department of Gynecology
University of Colorado
Denver, CO 80202

Division of Pediatric Surgery, Department of Surgery
Medical College of Virginia
Richmond, VA 23298

Division of Obstetrics
Prentice Women's Hospital & Maternity Center of
Northwestern Memorial Hospital
Chicago, IL 60611

Department of Obstetrics and Gynecology
Brigham and Women's Hospital
Boston, MA 02115

Division of Perinatal Medicine
Yale University School of Medicine
New Haven, CT 06510

Pregnancy Research Branch
National Institute of Mental Health
Bethesda, MD 20857

Why is a child like a chimney?

Because most of a youngster's body heat escapes through the top—of the head. So while a hat makes sense on a very cold day, the rest of the time you probably don't have to dress your child as warmly as you think.

Many mothers don't appreciate how snug a child can feel

because females have less tolerance for extremes of weather once they're old enough to bear children. But too many clothes can cause profuse sweating, and sweating often results in a chill, especially in cold weather.

Even in the worst weather, babies will do fine wearing a light sweater and a down-filled, moisture-repellent snowsuit over usual indoor clothing, plus lined boots and mittens—and that hat. By the way, if your youngster is allergic to wool or synthetics, try tying a large cotton kerchief around the child's head, under the hat. The cotton will prevent contact with sensitive skin.

Also, because babies can't usually communicate their discomfort, check to be sure yours isn't cold. Don't bother with the hands and feet; they're normally on the cool side. Instead, feel legs or arms or neck. If they're warm, so's your baby.

Mittens can be a nuisance, particularly when toddlers strip them off so they can use their hands better. Some strategies to outwit your recalcitrant mitten-stripper: Try extra-long ones and stuff them up into coat sleeves, sew them to the coat, or use Velcro fasteners or a short length of elastic or even large safety pins. Mittens are a must if the temperature dips below 25° F, according to Dr. William Cashore, a neonatologist at Women and Infants Hospital, Providence, Rhode Island. Frostbite is then a possibility. The mittens will also protect the child from direct contact with cold surfaces such as ice or concrete.

But take heart. By the time your child is four or five, Dr. Cashore says, he or she will probably appreciate mittens without coaxing.

What's as important as the ABCs?

Toddler gymnastics. Children who have learned coordination on the padded mat have, it's been discovered, a better feeling about themselves—and develop faster.

Even youngsters at the aptly named toddler stage can do simple gymnastic movements. It helps them develop coordination, balance, and body control—and they love it.

You can find preschool gymnastics programs in local recreation departments, Y's, colleges, and dancing schools, but often they don't welcome children under three. You can conduct your own classes at home, however. Of course, your child will not be ready to compete with Nadia Comaneci; toddler gymnastics are not like those for older children and adults, nor do they use the same equipment.

Here's how to do it yourself:

☐ Use a mat or a well-padded carpet, not a bed or bare floor. Dress yourself in loose clothing and don't wear shoes or jewelry. Remember that toddler back muscles are weak, and proceed gently.

☐ To train eye-hand and eye-foot coordination and motor skills, have the child throw a soft, large ball up in the air and catch it. Kick it back and forth. Roll the ball between your youngster's legs to teach beginning catch. After that's mastered, try regular catch, passing it gently to the child's hands after showing how to hold them.

☐ To teach concentration and provide a sense of movement, make a pattern on the floor with string. Start with a straight line and have your toddler walk along it. Then make it curvy. Pretend it's the yellow brick road.

☐ To improve concentration, devise a low balance beam by stretching a two-by-four on top of two bricks. At first, help your youngster walk across it, one foot in front of the other, by holding both hands. Then hold only one hand. Finally, let your budding gymnast try it alone, holding his or her arms outstretched for balance.

☐ Start to work on simple tumbling when your child becomes somewhat more coordinated. Some authorities say backward somersaults are a less scary way to begin than frontward ones. Show your child the starting position; that's easier than trying to explain it. Make sure your youngster's head is tucked between the legs. It makes the tumbling motion easier and prevents strain on the neck and back.

☐ Jumping and running are excellent exercises, too. Do them to music. Get your gymnast to jump over the balance beam, or jump back and forth across the string on the floor.

☐ Always keep your toddler's tender age and abilities in mind. Don't push. Be patient. Make it enjoyable for both of you.

Why is my son such a lazy student?

Are you sure he's really lazy? Educators and pediatricians estimate that between 10 and 15 percent of children with average or above-average IQs have one or more of a hundred learning disabilities—subtle physical impairments that make schoolwork very difficult for them. Three quarters of these children are boys; we don't know why.

Learning disabilities are recognized soon after the child begins school, or even before, although sometimes they are not apparent until early junior high, when the work becomes more complex. A recent study found that half of the adolescents labeled "lazy" turned out to have minor disabilities that blocked them from doing advanced math or writing a report.

In junior high, some children who did not find academic work particularly hard before now may develop difficulties in motor tasks, such as using a pen or pencil. Memory problems can express themselves in poor spelling, or trouble with rules of grammar and punctuation. Difficulties with written or spoken language are common, too. Such children are often impulsive; they cannot finish assignments, have trouble paying attention, and tend to ignore details. An affected child will commonly exhibit more than one of these symptoms. Because at this age saving face is all-important, he or she may try to disguise the problem, pretending indifference or acting defiant or hostile.

If your young child has a learning disability, make a special effort to read to the youngster, to talk and play, and in general to encourage learning. Provide a quiet, structured home where routine activities such as meals and bedtime come at predictable, regular hours.

Though schools in most states provide help, not all school systems that give special attention to younger children with learning disabilities make the same effort for older children. Nor are diagnostic techniques as far advanced for this age group. Parents, in collaboration with their pediatricians, may need to push harder to get help for their older child. One effective strategy combines remedial work with allowing a child to bypass some tasks—for example, permitting a youngster who writes with difficulty to tape-record a book report instead of writing it.

If your child is bright enough to handle school but is doing poorly, talk to his or her teacher and pediatrician. You can also get information from the following organizations:

Association for Children with Learning Disabilities
4156 Library Road
Pittsburgh, PA 15234

National Easter Seal Society
2023 W. Ogden Avenue
Chicago, IL 60612

Council for Exceptional Children
1920 Association Drive
Reston, VA 22091

National Institute of Mental Health
Public Inquiries Section
5600 Fishers Lane, Room 11A-19
Rockville, MD 20857

Orton Society
8415 Bellona Lane
Towson, MD 21204

Is your twelve-year-old too young for a pelvic exam?

Not if she complains of persistent pain in her lower abdomen.

When a young girl says she's having bad cramps you wonder if the problem might be emotional—her way of resisting impending womanhood—or maybe just too many French fries. The pediatrician has suggested it's functional, which means "I can't find anything wrong and it will probably go away."

Don't wait and wonder too long. Your daughter's trouble may be in her head or in her bowels, but it also may be in her uterus. If the pains don't go away, take her seriously and take her to a gynecologist.

According to Dr. Donald P. Goldstein, chief of gynecology at the Children's Hospital Medical Center in Boston and a faculty member of the Harvard Medical School, many pediatricians seem to be unaware of the relatively high incidence of gynecological disorders in teenagers. They often assume that pain associated with menstruation is psychological. But there are other reasons.

It is now known, for example, that overactivity of the prosta-glandins—body chemicals that stimulate uterine contractions—may contribute to severe menstrual cramps. If that's the problem, there are drugs that can help.

Pelvic pain may also stem from less common but more serious conditions. Dr. Goldstein reports that in a study of 201 young patients with distress chronic enough to warrant an exploratory procedure called laparoscopy, it was found that 48 percent had endometriosis, a condition in which cells from the lining of the uterus grow either within or outside the uterus. The condition can be treated, usually with drugs, if detected early.

The study also showed that 14 percent of the girls had pelvic lesions from previous abdominal surgery, and 5 percent had mal-formations of the uterus.

Some parents resist the idea of a pelvic examination for fear it will be upsetting to a young adolescent. This reluctance could cost your child unnecessary physical and mental anguish, and it might jeopardize her future reproductive health. Don't put off seeing the gynecologist.

When should you tell your daughter?

Well before menstruation begins—by the age of nine at least. That way the onset—when a girl turns into a woman—can be the time of joy it should be.

Of critical importance, no matter what the age, is knowing ahead of time what to expect. According to a survey, more than 36 percent of mothers tell their daughters little or nothing about menstruation, an omission that often causes the girl to be upset when it happens. What's more, how and when you tell her may affect how easily or painfully she experiences menstruation the rest of her life.

Don't be misled, either, by the old wisdom that your daughter will learn what she needs to know from schoolmates. It's better that she learn about it from you. And *how* you tell her is just as important as *what* you tell her. If you call menstruation "the curse" or something equally negative, your child's perception will obviously be colored. If, on the other hand, you convey that menarche introduces her to the wonder of womanhood, you will help her to appreciate and enjoy her own sexuality and identity throughout her life.

Experts suggest that nine is a good age to introduce the subject, which should be explained gradually, allowing time for questions, for reading, and for whatever else your child requires. This may seem a very young age to you, but about 10 percent of girls are menstruating by the age of ten.

And be specific about what you tell her—not clinical but clear about the physiological process, what organs are involved, how they relate to each other, where they are, and how she can expect them to function. This way, when you introduce her to the hygiene of menstruation, she will better understand what makes it necessary and not regard it as a way of getting rid of something unclean. Knowledge dispels fear.

By the way, education about menstruation is important for boys, too. Don't keep your son in the dark. His knowledge and resulting attitudes will bear directly on his attitudes toward women.

Is iodine too much of a good thing?

Apparently. Authorities—from the U.S. Food and Drug Administration and the American Medical Association, as well as Cornell University agricultural researchers—are finding that Americans may get too much iodine in their diets. Ironically, the overdose has come about because iodine deficiency was a major public-health problem early in this century.

The thyroid gland uses tiny amounts of dietary iodine to make the hormone that regulates body heat, assures healthy connective tissue, and is essential to physical and mental development. A thyroid gland starved for iodine tries to compensate by getting bigger. The resulting large swelling on the neck is called a goiter. It was common seventy-five years ago, but is virtually unknown today.

To prevent goiter, iodine was added to the American diet in a number of ways. The most familiar, iodized salt, first appeared in 1924. By the early 1970's, however, scientists had begun to realize that the pendulum was swinging in the other direction. An FDA study showed that a typical teenage boy was ingesting about five and a half times the recommended daily allowance for the mineral. The figures for young children were even higher. Toddlers were getting up to ten times the recommended intake, six-month-old babies up to thirteen times. Authorities were concerned because too much iodine is just as bad as too little. In fact, very large doses of iodine—much larger than those the FDA study has discovered—can lead to goiter, too.

Thanks to educational efforts by the government and medical groups, some food processors and dairy farmers have cut back their use of the mineral, but it can still creep into the body in unexpected ways. For example, pregnant and nursing women should avoid vaginal douches and gels containing povidone-iodine. The iodine can be absorbed in amounts high enough to harm a fetus, and it shows up in breast milk.

Other sources of iodine that are worth being cautious about include dairy products, which carry sanitizing iodophors that probably account for the high levels detected in young children, and sugars and sugary foods—jam, jelly, candy bars. Then, too, the use of Red Dye No. 3, which is 50 percent iodine, has almost doubled since two other food dyes were removed from the market in 1976. Its intake should be monitored to prevent excess, so read product labels carefully.

For most people who eat a lot of fish and dairy products, switching from iodized to plain salt is probably a good idea.

Does a fever mean you should call the pediatrician?

It depends on how high your child's temperature is and how long it's lasted. Not every situation requires pushing the panic button. Sometimes your caring will "cure" the ailment.

Basically, it's a case of common sense and using your parental instincts. An obvious medical emergency—a broken arm or leg, convulsions, breathing stoppage, serious bleeding—of course requires an immediate call for help. But most medical situations are subtler.

Although pediatricians' advice varies slightly, the younger your child, the quicker you should react. An illness or injury to a newborn baby, especially if accompanied by persistent vomiting or diarrhea, should be reported immediately.

Also consult the doctor if your child's general behavior and appearance change dramatically—for example, if a normally active child becomes lethargic, difficult to arouse, and incoherent, or if the child becomes unusually irritable or very pale and seems to be much sicker than usual.

Specific symptoms that warrant a phone call include:

- [ ] A temperature of 101 degrees persisting for more than one day. Call immediately, however, if a temperature of 104 degrees or higher does not respond to fever-lowering treatment.
- [ ] A severe cough that lasts more than twenty-four hours. This is especially true if the cough has a wheezing or barking quality. If there is serious difficulty in breathing—constant rapid breathing, blue lips, enlarged nostrils—call immediately.
- [ ] Bloody stools. Heavy bleeding requires an immediate call. Small amounts of streaking in stools should be watched and reported.
- [ ] Vomiting blood or green- or yellow-stained material.
- [ ] Vomiting combined with diarrhea when your child is unable to retain fluids for more than six hours.
- [ ] Any bleeding, especially nose bleeding.
- [ ] A gaping cut longer than one quarter inch.

Some persons feel shy about "bothering" their child's doctor, or are prone to listen to advice from friends. But there's no substitute for your own gut feelings. You know your child better than anyone else, and you have the advantage of being present on the scene. Phoning the doctor is often unnecessary. But if you *are* uncertain, trust your instincts. Don't hesitate to call.

Do lighting needs change with age?

Absolutely. Although almost a quarter of our population are now fifty or older, most lighting is designed for people in their twenties. Our eyes get short shrift—and we stumble our way into too many needless accidents.

As we get older most of us find it gets harder to see small

details up close, which is why we begin to need reading glasses after the age of forty or so. We may also find it more difficult to discriminate between subtle shades of colors, and we become less sensitive to contrasts between light and dark.

James L. Nuckolls, a lighting consultant, suggests the following ways to improve lighting in your home for both health and safety reasons:

- [ ] Eliminate glare by making sure lights are shielded even if they are not used for reading. Indirect glare from a highly polished floor, for example, creates optical illusions that lead to falls.
- [ ] Put lamps where they can illuminate particular activities, such as sewing or reading. In the kitchen, install fluorescent under-cabinet lighting close to work surfaces.
- [ ] Always locate switches and wall plates in the same place—the right-hand side, for example—and in convenient places, preferably near doorways. Luminous switches are a help.
- [ ] Illuminate stairs, doorsills, and other obstructions in the house and outdoors.
- [ ] Keep low-intensity lights on all the time in darkened areas—bedrooms, hallways, and bathrooms—to facilitate the eyes' adjustment to sudden changes from light to dark.
- [ ] Put light fixtures in closets in the front, either in the ceiling or on the side. But—and this holds true elsewhere as well—do not install fixtures so high that you have to stand on a chair or a step stool to change a bulb.

What's so good about mouthwash?

Very little, according to a recent study by a panel appointed by the Food and Drug Administration. The panel of experts checked out thirty-four ingredients used in mouthwashes and found that none of them was safe and effective. In fact, the panel recommended that ten of the ingredients—including boric acid, ferric chloride, potassium chlorate, sodium dichromate, phenol, and cetylpyridinium—should not be used at all.

Bad breath in the morning is something most people have,

but it doesn't indicate an oral disease. According to the FDA panel, most people can solve their breath problems by rinsing their mouths with water, brushing their teeth, flossing, or simply eating breakfast.

The experts not only discourage the use of antimicrobial ingredients in mouthwashes, they feel that advertisers should not claim on the label or in advertising that their products kill germs by the millions or in minutes, or that the mouthwash inhibits odor-forming bacteria.

In checking out products marketed for the temporary relief of sore throat, panel members found some ingredients acceptable, but they found no safe and effective ingredients that act as expectorants to remove thick secretions from the mouth and throat.

If you develop an oral condition that won't go away, it's best to consult your doctor or dentist rather than try a drugstore remedy. Similarly, if a sore throat becomes severe and persistent, see your doctor.

Need age preclude surgery?

A firm "No!" Particularly if you are one of the growing numbers of "young-old" people among us now. "Young-old" means you can be eighty plus but feel and behave like sixty or younger because you are in good physical shape and mental spirits.

On a single day, Dr. John C. Bowen III of New Orleans removed a woman's cancerous breast, took out another woman's gallbladder, and fixed a man's hernia. Not an unusual day's work for a surgeon, Arthur S. Freese wrote in *Modern Maturity* magazine, except that Dr. Bowen's three patients were respectively eighty-four, eighty-seven, and a hundred and three years old. Around the country, hundreds of thousands of operations are performed every year on men and women over sixty-five or seventy.

One hazard in older years is falling and breaking a hip bone that's become brittle with a condition called osteoporosis. That once meant being kept immobile, in a cast. But these days the treatment is prompt surgery to fix the hip in place with a metal pin, and a victim soon walks again. Last year more than 150,000 successful joint operations, mostly on hips and knees, were carried out on patients sixty or over. The reparative surgery should be carried out as soon as possible, experts say, then followed by rehabilitation and exercise programs.

As a surgical risk factor it isn't so much birthdays that count as how well a person has taken care of himself or herself. Learning someone's chronological age is easy—birth certificates and other documents count the years—but judging physiological age is different. How does a person look? How active is he or she in daily living?

There are tips on how to limit the risks of elective (non-emergency) surgery for older people. If you have chronic lung disease, schedule the operation in spring or summer, when respiratory infections are less common, suggests Dr. Tom J. Wachtel of Providence, Rhode Island, writing in the journal *Geriatrics.* He also advises having the surgery later in the day, in order to give a patient who may have bronchitis or emphysema time to clear his or her respiratory passages in the morning.

Some experts on aging suggest that if a doctor or surgeon turns you down for pain-relieving or restorative surgery just because of birthdays, you should get a second opinion.

What's a good reason to feed an infant while in your arms?

The position can help to prevent otitis media. This infant ailment, known as middle-ear disease, is very common. Almost one third of all babies born in the United States contract it before their first birthday. The symptom is earache, and because it affects hearing, the earache could affect a baby's development.

Doctors have not yet pinpointed to their satisfaction the cause of middle-ear disease. But according to a recent article in *Medical Times,* most doctors attribute it to improper functioning of an infant's eustachian tube. The tube in an adult is at a fairly acute angle, allowing for normal drainage of secretions. But the muscle that controls the eustachian tube does not begin to function efficiently in a person until after puberty, and the cartilage of the eustachian tube is soft in infants. Consequently, in an infant the tube is constantly collapsed and almost horizontal, and the muscle opens only with difficulty. The horizontal position increases the secretions in the inner ear, which build up in the collapsed tube. The situation is aggravated because infants spend so much time lying down.

Because they're usually fed while in a horizontal position, bottle-fed babies get middle-ear disease more often than breast-fed babies. This is especially so for infants whose bottles are propped so that they drink while on their backs, because swallowing when lying down allows bacteria to travel from the mouth and nose into the ear.

If you're a new mother, whether breast-feeding or bottle-feeding, hold your baby sitting up in your arms. You will help prevent middle-ear disease, and you will give your baby important emotional nourishment as well.

One more caution: Other factors occasionally cause middle-ear disease, inducing staph infections, even pneumonia. So if you think your baby has an earache, begin the cure with a call to your pediatrician.

Is your baby safe and secure?

Probably not. There are many hazards lurking in baby equipment, and many precautions you as a parent should take, beginning with the cradle. Make certain the cradle is solid and can't tip over. The mattress should fit snugly against the sides, so that your infant's head can't get caught.

Don't keep your baby in the cradle too long; it's unsafe once the baby starts turning over. Then it's time to switch to a crib—still exercising caution. As the U.S. Consumer Product Safety Commission estimates, between 150 and 200 children under two years old die every year in crib accidents, and 40,000 more are hurt badly enough to need a doctor's care. Many of them suffocate between the mattress and the crib sides. Others catch their heads between crib slats that are too wide. Some fall out of cribs with sides too low, or swing out of cribs with horizontal bars. The commission warns against using a Starlighter crib, made by a now-bankrupt firm. The firm refused to recall or repurchase the cribs after a baby died of asphyxiation when she caught her head between the slats.

Since 1974 crib makers have had to meet certain safety requirements, but they have not been required since 1976 to display labels showing that their cribs meet the requirements. As a rule of thumb:

- [ ] The crib slats should be no more than 2⅜ inches apart. (That's about three adult fingers.)
- [ ] The crib sides should be no less than 26 inches high from the bottom of the mattress to the top of the rail.
- [ ] When the drop side is down, it should measure at least 9 inches high from the top of the mattress.
- [ ] Horizontal bars, which could be steps for climbing out, should be avoided.
- [ ] Crib sides should lock at their maximum height.
- [ ] The drop side's latching device should not release easily.
- [ ] Wood surfaces should be splinter-free, metal hardware have smooth edges, paint be nontoxic.
- [ ] Bumper pads (useful to separate baby from crib slats) should fasten or tie in at least six places.
- [ ] Decorative cutouts are not desirable. Current specifications are unsafe and are being revised by the commission.

In addition, if more than two adult fingers can fit between a mattress and the crib sides, it is too loose. Replace it or stuff tightly rolled towels, too big for a baby to pull loose, in the space around the mattress edge.

The rules for choosing a portable crib are similar, with these exceptions:

- [ ] Crib sides should be no less than 22 inches from mattress bottom to railing top.
- [ ] The distance between mattress top and rail top when the drop side is down should be no less than 5 inches.
- [ ] Latches on folding sides should require at least ten pounds of force to open and close or should require two separate actions.

The Consumer Products Safety Commission suggests that a crib is too small when the side rail is less than three quarters of the child's height. A portable crib is too small after the child has grown to thirty-five inches. Then it's bed time.

As for playpens, there are two basic kinds, the traditional model with criblike wooden slats and the newer one with a padded frame supporting mesh sides. The following guidelines should apply:

☐ The slats of a slatted playpen should be no farther apart than 2⅜ inches, or three adult fingers, the same as the crib measurements.

☐ Make certain the floor is flat and firm, otherwise it could collapse when the baby is standing.

☐ The hinges of the folding model should lock tightly and have no sharp edges.

☐ The mesh weave should be too small to catch baby buttons or be used as a ladder for climbing out.

Safety gates can be dangerous, too, because children can injure themselves trying to climb over them and falling, catching their necks. If you plan to use one, install it in a climb-proof place.

When it comes to infant walkers, some experts believe they are so dangerous that they caution against having one. A recent study of 150 children between five and fifteen months old showed that over a three-month period 31 percent hurt themselves using walkers. Most of the injuries were minor cuts and bruises, but several were serious—including skull fractures and a tooth ripped out badly enough to require dental surgery.

By the way, the walker is supposed to speed up learning to walk, but another study shows that, if anything, the reverse is true. The babies who didn't use walkers at all walked slightly sooner than the babies who did.

The Consumer Products Safety Commission has other safety information about children's equipment. Call its hotline toll-free, (800) 638-8326; in Maryland, (800) 492-8363; in Alaska, Hawaii, Puerto Rico, and the Virgin Islands, (800) 638-8333.

What's the new miracle drug in your pantry?

Would you believe sugar? Doctors are finding that this sweet substance can help to speed the healing of wounds, burns, and skin ulcers. Moreover, it is safe, cheap, easy to get and to use.

In Argentina, scientists at the University of Buenos Aires

packed the infected wounds of 120 patients with ordinary granulated sugar and found in 99 percent of the cases that the bacterial infections cleared in nine days to seventeen weeks. In the United States, doctors at the Delta Medical Center in Greenville, Mississippi, have reported similar success in a five-year study involving 605 patients suffering from wounds, skin ulcers, and burns.

The Greenville doctors say the therapy, a combination of sugar and povidone-iodine, a mild anti-infective agent, "outperforms all other products for wound care and is the combination we most depend upon for wound, burn, or ulcer treatment." They found that wounds so treated healed faster than with alternative standard therapy, and with little or no scarring. The need for antibiotics was reduced, as was the reliance on painkillers—dressings can simply be washed off with water.

Sugar works its wonders in several ways. It is naturally antibacterial, inhibiting the growth of microorganisms. It soaks up moisture and thus helps reduce the swelling common to injured tissue. Sugar may also provide the nourishment or stimulus for tissue to regenerate.

One word of caution: When using sugar, make sure that bleeding from a wound has stopped for twenty-four hours before applying.

Today's observations only confirm the wisdom of ancient practice. As early as 1700 B.C. Egyptian physicians were touting the benefits of packing battlefield wounds with a mixture of grease and sugar-rich honey. We don't advise that, but the more things change . . .

Why would you ever want to bite on a cork?

To stop a nosebleed.

Ruptures of the tiny blood vessels inside the nose are responsible for most nosebleeds, but you don't have to engage in fisticuffs to get them. They can result from something as minor as sneezing or blowing your nose.

You can often stop the bleeding yourself by pinching your nostrils between finger and thumb, while applying ice to the bridge of your nose. If this doesn't work, hold a small bowl under your nose to catch the blood while you wait for a clot to form. Try not to swallow, because that will displace the clot. Gripping a cork between your teeth will keep you from swallowing. Allow your saliva to drip into the bowl.

In addition, the *British Medical Journal* advises that the position of your body can be important in stemming the bleeding. Younger people who have lost only a little blood can stay upright, but older people, or those who have lost a lot of blood, should keep their heads low.

One thing you shouldn't do is pack the nostril with cotton or tissue. That only keeps the broken blood vessels open.

If bleeding persists, get to a hospital. Doctors might want to spray your nose with medication to constrict the blood vessels.

Can kids get migraines?

Surprisingly enough, they can. And they're not as rare as we used to think. In fact, about one third of recurring headaches among children are that throbbing "sick headache" called migraine. At what age do they begin? As young as a year old, but they are more common among older children and teenagers.

As those who suffer from migraine know, the agonizing pain of this headache is something special, and is accompanied by other symptoms as well, most often nausea and vomiting. The headache itself results from dilation of the arteries in the head, although it is usually preceded by constriction of those arteries, which causes other symptoms, such as the "aura" (blurred vision, flashing lights) that often alerts the sufferer to a headache on the way. No one knows exactly what causes the arteries to narrow and then widen in this way.

Migraine is apparently a genetic disorder. If you get migraines, there's a 60 percent chance your children will eventually develop them too, and the chances may rise to better than 80 percent if your spouse is a fellow sufferer.

Children's migraines differ somewhat from those of adults. They usually get the so-called common migraine, in which there is no well-defined aura. But they may complain of feeling dizzy or sick to their stomachs as the headache progresses, and will frequently be very pale.

What causes migraines? Experts agree that the leading trigger is stress, which is often related to emotional problems at school, peer relations, or family difficulties. Some sufferers react to certain foods, especially chocolate and cheeses. Teenage girls may find attacks coming on with their menstrual periods, or if they begin using a contraceptive pill.

Can anything be done for childhood migraines? Happily, yes. First, make sure your child's headaches really are migraines; children get recurring headaches for many reasons. Your pediatrician can usually diagnose the cause of the youngster's headaches, although in some cases the doctor may advise seeing a specialist in pediatric neurology.

Although strong and effective drugs are available, the experts say that they should be a last resort in children's migraines because of their side effects. The first line of defense is prevention: Identify and remove the factors that trigger the attacks. If problems at school or at home seem to be responsible, find a way to resolve the difficulties. If lack of sleep or irregular eating patterns are implicated, get your child on a regular schedule and enforce it.

Migraines can be treated effectively with plain aspirin or other simple analgesics, combined with rest in a darkened room. The headache and other symptoms can frequently be headed off altogether if treatment comes at the beginning of an attack, so teach your child to pay attention to warning symptoms and to take aspirin and lie down right away when they occur. Some doctors believe that biofeedback and relaxation techniques can be mastered and used successfully by children of ten or older. If these measures fail, your child's pediatrician may want to consider prescribing medication.

What's likely to bite the hand that feeds it?

A dog, of course. And in 80 percent of reported dog bites it was most probably a family dog or a neighbor's dog.

Dr. Alan M. Beck, director of the Center for the Interaction of Animals and Society at the University of Pennsylvania's School of Veterinary Medicine, also found that more than 60 percent of reported dog bites happen between July and September, that the most frequent victims are boys under the age of fifteen, and that they are most frequently bitten by shepherds and similar large male dogs.

At least a million people each year are treated for dog bites, at a cost of over $50 million, and it's estimated that at least another million cases go unreported. To avoid bites and to train your child to do so:

- [ ] Don't put your face near a dog's face.
- [ ] Assume that any barking or snarling dog will bite.
- [ ] Don't look it in the eye. Turn sideways. Call sharply, something like "Go home," to startle the dog and fend off the attack.
- [ ] Don't move or shout suddenly.
- [ ] Never bother a dog—even lovingly—by touching it when it's eating or sleeping.
- [ ] Keep hands off strange dogs. If one approaches, train your child to stand still, hands at sides. Try not to frighten the dog.

If you are bitten, the likelihood is that you won't get rabies, which is rare in the United States. Yet each year there are more than thirty thousand rabies treatments started, about ten times what the Centers for Disease Control in Atlanta estimates is necessary. So if you're bitten, first identify the dog and determine if it's been vaccinated against rabies. If you can't and there has been rabies in your area, you will probably need the series of rabies shots. In addition, if you're bitten:

- [ ] Flush the wound with plenty of soap and warm water.
- [ ] See a doctor, either your own or one in the nearest emergency room. Even if the dog isn't rabid, dog bites are serious. The risk of infection from them is very high; there are some sixty-five different bacteria in a dog's mouth that can infect humans. Dog's teeth are strong enough to cut sheet metal.

But don't let all this talk of injury dampen your decision to buy a dog. Experts who've studied animal-human relations say that dogs are excellent companions for children and aged people.

For the aged, dogs can ease loneliness; for children, owning a dog can promote empathy, self-control, self-esteem, and a sense of responsibility.

But keep a few things in mind when you're choosing a dog. First, you'd better think of the pet as a ten-year commitment, and like a child that doesn't grow up, it requires care and attention as long as it lives. Then consider the following:

- ☐ Size and breed. Experts think mixed breeds make the best pets, but if you want a full breed, choose a gentle one. A large percentage of dog bites are blamed on shepherds and shepherd mixes.
- ☐ Wait to buy a dog until your child is five years old. A study at the University of Chicago's Wyler Children's Hospital showed that children four years old and under were bitten more frequently by the family dog than were older children. Half a million children under five are bitten by dogs every year.
- ☐ Look for a curious pup. Shy ones might be nervous and grow up to be biters. Growling pups should be passed up.
- ☐ If you get your dog from an animal shelter, you not only get it free or for nominal charge, you may get free neutering or spaying, shots, and follow-up care for thirty days.
- ☐ If you buy your dog, have it checked thoroughly by a veterinarian within the first four or five days.
- ☐ Train the dog—and its owner. Some animal shelters offer training courses for $50 or less.

Is there a way to treat male infertility?

Yes, in some cases. Menotropins (Pergonal), a drug already successful in overcoming infertility in women, has now been approved for men by the Food and Drug Administration.

Traditionally, when a couple is unable to have a baby the woman gets tested first, despite the fact that it's a fifty-fifty chance that it's the man's problem. And tests for men are relatively quick, easy, painless, and inexpensive, much more so than for women—so the difficulty in conception can often be corrected faster if the man is tested first.

For thousands of men the problem is a pituitary deficiency that results in decreased production of sperm. (The jawbreaking medical name for the condition is hypogonadotropic hypogonadism.) Specifically, the pituitary, the body's master gland, fails to secrete either one or both of two hormones—luteinizing hormone and follicle-stimulating hormone—both of which are present in men and women.

Menotropins has been so successful that some women using it had multiple births—twins and triplets. Men in twenty-five countries outside the United States already use it.

Tests on men in this country since 1974 have shown that more than 75 percent with this condition who took the drug were able to father children. The sperm counts of some being treated reached effective levels in six to nine months, according to the National Institute of Child Health and Human Development. Six months of treatment is estimated to cost about $1,400.

There are other developments in fertility treatment besides menotropins. For example, the most common cause of male infertility, varicocele, which is caused by a varicose vein in the scrotum, is now treatable in many men, either through surgery or by means of devices inserted into the scrotum. So if a couple has been attempting to conceive for more than a year (six months if the woman is over thirty), both wife and husband should see the doctor.

What can save a senior citizen's eyesight?

The fabulous light beam known as a laser, which can be harnessed to become a precise surgical knife within the delicate eye itself.

Lasers are now saving the sight of many elderly people who develop a vision problem known as senile neovascular macular degeneration—the overgrowth of tiny blood vessels into a part of the eye called the macula. Only as big as a thumbtack, the macula controls central vision in the retina, or screen of the eye. Excessive blood vessel growth can cause bleeding, scar formation, and retinal damage, impairing vision.

By one estimate, about one third of the men and women over age sixty are at risk of macular degeneration. The problem affects women more than men, and is more common among people with blue eyes and light coloring; it is rare among black people. The degeneration may not cause serious damage, but the excessive growth of abnormal blood vessels—which occurs in 10 percent of patients with senile macular degeneration—can cause blindness unless checked. Researchers estimate that if the trouble were detected soon enough, as many as 13,000 older Americans would not go blind each year.

People over fifty can perform a simple test for macular degeneration: Pick out a straight line—a doorframe or telephone pole, for example. Cover one eye and see if the line is still straight, then check the other eye. If the line appears bent or distorted or if a blank spot appears, the National Eye Institute advises, an ophthalmologist should be seen immediately. The laser treatment to cure it is painless and takes only about ten minutes.

The use of lasers is also beneficial in the treatment of diabetic retinopathy, the leading cause of adult blindness in the United States, affecting more than 300,000 people twenty to sixty-four years old each year. Until now, the Hospital of the University of Pennsylvania discovered, signs of the eye disease have been missed in more than 60 percent of all cases by doctors who treat diabetics.

Because the cause of retinopathy is unclear and the disease doesn't become clinically apparent for years, the hospital says that the symptoms can best be diagnosed by an ophthalmologist—and that people who have had diabetes for a number of years should have regular eye checkups. Laser treatment, the National Eye Institute reports, can reduce the risk of blindness by 50 percent or more.

What may be risky for flu or chickenpox?

Quite possibly, that favorite fever fighter—aspirin. A controversy is raging in medical circles about the connection between aspirin and a disease known as Reye's Syndrome. The U.S. Surgeon General, for one, insists aspirin can do more harm than good if given to children who have either the flu or chickenpox.

Reye's Syndrome—a rare and puzzling collection of signs, symptoms, and physical effects—usually develops in a youngster who gets a virus infection, notably influenza or chickenpox, and is given aspirin to bring down the fever. In one study, 97 percent of the youngsters who developed the syndrome had taken aspirin to fight off chickenpox and flu.

A child who develops Reye's Syndrome becomes irritable and confused; hands may feel clammy, eyes appear glazed. If the disease is not caught in time, the child may have lingering mental retardation as a result of brain damage, or, in a few cases, die. Fortunately, if it is diagnosed early, the chances of recovery are good.

No one knows why Reye's Syndrome develops in some children with virus infections, or why aspirin—usually beneficial—might contribute to the disease. There is speculation that aspirin somehow blocks absorption of vitamin C.

Even though there is disagreement that aspirin is the culprit in Reye's Syndrome, many experts are now advising caution in using it for flu and chickenpox. It's no fun having either of those ailments, but they are usually not life-threatening. A mild to moderate fever caused by a virus infection can be treated by sponging the body with tepid water, and there are substitute drugs for aspirin.

What should you look out for after menopause?

Iron. Some women may have too much of it. And that, according to a recent study, may induce some types of heart disease, because an excess of iron can cause irregular heartbeat and disorders of the heart muscle.

A woman is relatively better protected than a man against heart disease until after menopause. Two things happen at that time: Estrogen levels drop and iron is no longer lost in her monthly menstrual cycle. That usually removes the need for iron supplements. The situation, however, is not that simple. Tens of thousands of elderly women eat so sparingly that they require iron supplements to avoid iron-deficiency anemia.

After menopause, be certain you're eating a balanced diet. If it is balanced, meat consumption can be limited to three ounces three times a week, because meat is high in iron. And more fibrous foods and cereals can be added, because they absorb iron.

But don't decide on your own what to do. Let your doctor assess your needs.

Who knows all about medications?

Not just the doctor who prescribes them. A well-trained, conscientious pharmacist usually knows more about drugs than some physicians do, which is why choosing a good pharmacist is important to your health.

The most common form of medical treatment today is drugs. We benefit from an enormous number of medicines that save us from once life-threatening ailments. But many of these drugs are potentially toxic. Adverse drug reactions, which cost many lives and millions of dollars a year, are almost always foreseeable and preventable.

Doctors sometimes forget to ask patients about allergies or other conditions that might affect reactions to a drug, or may not know about these reactions. A conscientious pharmacist will ask for a medical history and inform you if you are in danger of a bad reaction.

Some people take different drugs at the same time, prescribed by different doctors for different conditions, without realizing each doctor should be told so. A good pharmacist keeps a record of your prescriptions and informs you and your doctors if you are in danger of harmful drug interaction.

Then, too, it's common for patients, nervous in the doctor's office, to forget what they've been told about the dosage and timing of medication. A good pharmacist will go over these instructions and write them clearly on the drug package, and will also remind you if there are substances—alcohol, for example—that you should avoid while under medication.

The question many people have about whether to purchase a generic or a brand-name drug seems rhetorical—both contain the same basic ingredient, and the generic one is always less expensive. However, there are cases in which different materials used to fill out a pill, such as the coloring or the coating, can affect what is called "bioavailability"—that is, the degree to which the active ingredient gets into your bloodstream. The pharmacist can usually answer your questions about which to purchase by consulting guides issued by the Food and Drug Administration. If you need to take medicine for a chronic condition over a long period of time, generic drugs, provided they are of proven effectiveness, can save you a small fortune.

When you find a good pharmacy, remember that it will sometimes be closed. Find out what emergency pharmacy facilities are available in the neighborhood for those times. Remember, too, that the best drugstore in the neighborhood isn't necessarily the most expensive one. Don't be afraid to shop around.

The University of Southern California School of Pharmacy will send you its publication "How to Select a Family Pharmacist" if you send a stamped, self-addressed envelope to Communications Committee, U.S.C. School of Pharmacy, 1985 Zonal Avenue, Suite 102, Los Angeles, CA 90033.

Meanwhile, for the fun of it, here's a quickie guide to those chicken scrawls—actually Latin or Latin abbreviations—on your prescription:

Rx	prescription
ac	before meals
ad lib	freely as needed
bid	twice daily
c	with
cap	capsule
gtt	a drop
hs	at bedtime
one tablet q.i.d.	one tablet four times a day

—————————————
——————

Should your child's tonsils come out?

Not necessarily. A tonsillectomy could be harmful for a child, because tonsils are a vital part of the immune system.

A major study of the operation's possible effects was undertaken in the 1970s at the University of Pittsburgh. One important feature of the research was that all the children studied had had several bouts of serious throat infection. Yet nearly half the children who did not have an operation did almost as well as those who did have it. The authors of the study concluded that the benefits of most tonsillectomies are questionable and that the operation should be performed only in special cases.

As a result of this and other studies, tonsillectomy went from being the most common major operation as late as 1971 to the third most common more recently. Yet there are still 600,000 tonsillectomies performed each year, and probably more than half are unnecessary.

So if your doctor recommends a tonsillectomy, be sure to seek a second opinion.

The operation may be recommended for the following reasons:

1. If serious bouts of tonsillitis have occurred seven times in one year, or five times a year for two years, or three times a year for three years. "Serious" means that the tonsillitis includes one or more of the following characteristics: enlarged glands in the neck; high fever; the presence of pus; or a positive strep culture, indicating the presence of an infection-causing type of *Streptococcus* bacteria.

2. If the tonsils are so large that the child's breathing is obstructed for six months or longer, because that can lead to heart and lung problems. Adenoids that are obstructive should be removed as well. But both those situations are rare.

The same rules apply to adult tonsillectomy. If the tonsils become a source of chronic infection, they should be removed. About 20 percent of the tonsillectomies performed at the Yale University Medical School are done on adults who have had at least seven serious infections in a single year.

But not all adult "tonsillitis" may really be tonsillitis. A study published in the *Archives of Otolaryngology* disclosed that fourteen patients who appeared to have recurring throat-and-tonsil infections actually suffered from common allergies to substances found in the air, such as plant pollens, animal dander, and house dust. If you suffer infections, it might be wise to have yourself tested for allergies before agreeing to an operation.

Does your baby care if you can carry a tune?

A Pavarotti or a Sills you don't have to be. If you're a new mother, your baby recognizes your voice only two or three days after birth—and loves it no matter how tuneless it sounds.

What's more, you're not only soothing the baby with your

lullaby, you're cementing your relationship as well. When you sing, the baby coos back at you, and those coos prompt you to love and care for the baby more. "It is a circle," say Dr. John Lind, professor emeritus at the Karolinska Institute in Stockholm, Sweden, and Carol Hardgrove, associate clinical professor of family health care nursing at the University of California, San Francisco. "Parent croons, the infant responds, the parent feels more parental, the infant feels more secure." In addition, you're providing the baby with important early language training.

Babies enjoy recorded instrumental and vocal music, but it doesn't reinforce the bond between the two of you the way a lullaby does. Lind and Hardgrove think singing to the baby is so important that they recommend women begin while they're still pregnant. Fetuses can hear in the womb, and many mothers-to-be claim that singing has a calming effect on the fetus during pregnancy as well as on the newborn infant.

As you sing, don't forget to rock your baby. Scientists have confirmed what your grandmother knew: Rocking is not only fun for babies, it's good for them. Studies on premature infants have shown that those who are rocked have a larger head circumference and better body coordination, visual and hearing responses, and weight gain than preemies who are not rocked. Full-term babies profit as well. Research shows that normal infants who are subjected to motion sit up and learn head control earlier than those who are not.

Why? Motion probably teaches a baby about the relationship between the body and the rest of the world. "Motion is important in the maintenance and development of all motor and neurological systems in a baby's body," says Mary V. Neal, chairman of the Department of Maternal and Child Nursing at the University of Maryland, who conducted some of the research on preemies. Scientists believe being deprived of motion can cause degeneration of nerve pathways in the infant brain.

Neal thinks hospital nurseries should regard rocking chairs as standard equipment, and so should households with a new baby. But the comfortable, old-fashioned rocker isn't the only way to provide the motion that's so necessary to child development. Just carrying the baby—in your arms, on your hip, or against your chest in one of those newfangled cloth carriers—works too. Babies usually enjoy swings and jumpers, but the equipment alone doesn't provide the variety of stimulating motions a baby gets from being carried by a loving parent.

Is Mother's cooking really better than store-bought baby foods?

Not necessarily, especially if you add salt. Salt in the diet is suspected of contributing to high blood pressure, the serious health problem that affects as many as one in every three persons. Some scientists think a high salt intake during infancy means greater susceptibility to high blood pressure later in life.

The problem becomes acute because, as one study discovered, homemade baby food ordinarily contains *ten times* as much salt as the supermarket kind. (Commercial baby-food manufacturers stopped adding salt to their products after being alerted to the problem.)

If fixing homemade food for your baby is important to you, by all means go ahead—but don't add salt, and don't use prepared ingredients such as canned vegetables that contain salt.

When is a good girl too good?

When it's more appropriate to be bad.

Psychologists tell us that all young children, but especially girls around the age of five or six, have a tough time reconciling the good and bad urges within them. "Our society," Dr. Joan Costello of the University of Chicago notes, "values girls—or women—primarily when they are good and self-controlled, whereas it permits and forgives a certain amount of brashness and rashness in boys—and men."

The tightly controlled little girl is afraid that any sign of self-assertiveness or misconduct may deny her approval and love. She's *too* good, unable to accept her own "naughty" feelings and secretly believing that she's really not good enough.

Research has shown that girls generally have lower expectations for themselves and less persistence in overcoming difficulties than boys do, even though girls generally start out way ahead of boys academically. What happens as they approach the high school and college years?

In one study, psychologists found that boys and girls interpret teacher evaluation differently. The boys felt that a poor evaluation of their performance represented a negative view both of their behavior and of their intellectual ability, and that correction of the former would improve the latter. The girls, on the other hand, were more debilitated by failure, much less likely to feel they could eventually be successful. They viewed their failure as a valid comment on their intellectual ability and believed that no effort on their part could change matters.

Dr. Costello, for one, feels strongly that parents should recognize that all children—girls as well as boys—need to learn how to balance being good and bad. "The long-term consequences of being too good too early," she says, "can only indicate that we should allow a little bit of brattiness in our children."

So let her act bratty once in a while. You don't have to like it—but be sure she knows you still love her, angel or not.

Is there a drug-free future for epileptics?

Indeed yes, for many of the millions of children with epilepsy. The possibility depends on whether the child has had epilepsy for a long time before seizure control and the type of disorder suffered.

Epilepsy is classified in three major categories: grand mal, the "big" seizure in which victims fall unconscious; petit mal, the "little" seizure, which may be no more than a short and slight spell of inattention; and psychomotor epilepsy, with its bizarre behavior, again for a short time.

Today, 80 percent of Americans with epilepsy have their disease controlled by effective anticonvulsant drugs. But while the drugs do wonders, there are impressive findings that they needn't be continued forever. The latest evidence is a long-term study by Dr. Jean Holowach Thurston and associates of Washington University School of Medicine and St. Louis Children's Hospital. In 1950 they began a study of 148 children with epilepsy whose seizures had long been controlled by drugs for a four-year period. The children were gradually taken off medication. By 1966, only about 25 percent of them had suffered a recurrence. Those with psychomotor epilepsy or who suffered a combination of seizure types were most susceptible to a relapse.

Dr. Thurston's team pushed on further, keeping tabs on the "kids" for fifteen to twenty-three years longer. They found that 41 of the 148—only 28 percent of them—had a recurrence of seizures. By then, some of the seizure-free patients had reached the age of forty.

Knowing a child's type and history of seizure, Dr. Thurston says, can help guide physicians in deciding when it is safe to recommend reducing the youngster's medication. Talk to your doctor if you think your child might benefit from this approach.

In the meantime, if a seizure occurs, experts now advise that you do *not* try to force a hard object between the epileptic's teeth. They say it's a myth that a person can swallow his or her tongue. What's more likely to occur is that the person will choke or swallow the object. Medical assistance is not necessary unless the seizure lasts more than fifteen minutes or a series of grand mal–type attacks occur in rapid succession.

What three initials can be dangerous?

Unless used with care, PPA. They stand for a name so long that it's easier to swallow than to say—phenylpropanolamine. It's one of the key ingredients in nonprescription weight-loss preparations, used often in combination with caffeine. It's also used in many cold remedies to help unclog stuffy noses. It acts like amphetamine (speed).

In 1981, estimates were that some 4 million people were taking some 10 billion doses of PPA annually. Increasingly, experts feel that it is a potentially dangerous drug, especially when combined with caffeine. A large percentage of the diet pills on the market now join PPA and caffeine. And there is evidence that when amphetamines are unavailable, this combination is being sold illegally as an "upper."

In 1982, there were at least ten thousand reports of PPA poisoning, a thousand of which required medical care. The patients' symptoms included hypertension, anxiety, agitation, hallucinations, hyperventilation, excessively rapid breathing, strokes, and intracerebral hemorrhages. Doses of PPA were as small as 50 to 75 milligrams, and with or without caffeine.

Many experts think that such diet aids are virtually useless. If you still want to use them, at least take these precautions:

☐ Don't use the weight-loss preparation for longer than three months, and only to lose weight. If you use it to maintain weight you could overuse it.

☐ Don't use more than the recommended dosage.

☐ Check with your doctor before using one if you have high blood pressure, heart disease, diabetes, or thyroid disease, if you're being treated for depression, or if you're already using a drug with PPA.

☐ Be very careful if you use a drug with PPA and caffeine and you still drink coffee, colas, tea, or other caffeine-filled liquids. Too much caffeine can make you sick.

☐ Don't let your children near PPA. All the symptoms are intensified in children.

☐ Be on the lookout for hidden PPA, which is often found in cough and cold remedies. If you're taking diet pills *and* a cold remedy, you could be getting an overdose.

☐ If you overdose, call your doctor, a poison control center, or the nearest hospital. Don't try to treat yourself.

Can garlic protect from anything but vampires?

Decidedly. It could be a nemesis of heart disease.

When oil of garlic—the juice—was given to healthy volunteers and to people who had previously had heart attacks, it seemed to significantly reduce blood levels of cholesterol and triglycerides. An ounce a day, it was found, may help protect against atherosclerosis, the narrowing of heart arteries due to fatty deposits or plaques, which contain the cholesterol and triglycerides.

While it hasn't entirely been proven that cholesterol and triglycerides trigger heart attacks, most physicians agree there is a strong link. They advise middle-aged and older people to restrict the consumption of foods high in them.

According to Dr. Arun Bordia, reporting in the *American Journal of Clinical Nutrition*, garlic seems to prevent blood cells from clumping together to form dangerous clots in the arteries feeding the heart.

There is also a bonus in using garlic—either minced raw or in oil of garlic capsules sold by many health-food stores. You can use it to season food and then skip the use of salt. High salt use is associated with high blood pressure, which is one of the principal risk factors linked to heart disease.

By the way, garlic may have value in fighting another major disease. Chinese doctors report that eating several cloves of garlic a day may protect against gastric cancer by lowering the amount of nitrites, which are believed to be cancer-forming substances in gastric juices.

Incidentally, if you're worried about bad breath, chomp a sprig of parsley afterward. It's a natural breath freshener.

What's one way to keep fit as a fiddle?

Dance to one. Folk dancing is fun—and also terrific exercise.

In a recent study of the benefits of an energetic Swedish folk dance known as the *hambo,* carried out at that country's National Board of Occupational Safety and Health, scientists discovered just how terrific. They tested six female and six male *hambo* dancers between the ages of twenty-two and thirty-two. While dancing, the men used an average of 70 percent of the maximum amount of oxygen their bodies were able to take in. (This is known as aerobic power. Exercise that uses more than 60 percent of aerobic power is usually thought to achieve the "training effect." It increases fitness, strengthening in particular the heart and lungs.) The effect for women was even greater; they used an average of 90 percent of their aerobic power.

In boosting fitness, folk dancing has a training effect similar to that of aerobic dancing, currently a popular and trendy pursuit for people eager to get in shape and stay there. Doctors caution, however, that while vigorous dancing can be healthy, it's important to know your limits. Join in carefully at first, especially if you haven't exercised for a while. Dancing as part of a group is so exhilarating that it's easy to overdo without realizing it. In fact, if you're well into your thirties or older, check with your doctor before starting, especially if you're out of shape.

For most people, dancing, whether folk or aerobic, has other benefits, too: It doesn't cost much, it's simple to learn and do, and it can be done year round. So if you've been looking for a good aerobic exercise but jogging isn't your thing, find a folk-dance group in your community and spend a few evenings a week enjoying jigs and polkas and turkey-in-the-straw.

What do maturity and misery have in common?

Sometimes, milk.

Pity the poor fellow who gulps a glass of cold milk on a hot afternoon. Pretty soon he has gas, stomach cramps, and diarrhea, and it never occurs to him (or, probably, to his doctor) that the culprit is milk. After all, milk didn't make him sick when he was ten years old.

The answer may be something called lactase deficiency. Lactase is an enzyme that facilitates the digestion of a sugar (lactose) that is a key ingredient of milk and milk products. If this sugar is not properly digested it causes an increase in intestinal bacteria, which in turn cause gas, stomach cramps, even diarrhea. Most children manufacture all the lactase they need. But for some unexplained reason, the production of lactase declines dramatically in 30 million adults. And because lactose is so common in so many foods—breads, cakes, cereals—and is also an ingredient in many common drugs, doctors often overlook lactase deficiency as the cause of stomach trouble.

It would seem obvious that the best way to cure the problem is to avoid milk and milk products. But the old wisdom that you need a quart of milk a day to keep your bones and teeth strong and to prevent bone loss may be true for many of us.

So what's the alternative? Warming the milk makes it easier to digest. Try creamed soups, and cultured milk products like yogurt, buttermilk, sour cream, and most cheeses. They contain bacteria that also speed the process of lactose digestion.

If that doesn't help, there are nonprescription preparations such as LactAid, which predigest lactose, that can be purchased at a drugstore. They can be added easily to milk or ice cream.

If you've been suffering from chronic stomach problems associated with milk consumption, it's worth trying these remedies. However, if the problem continues, obviously it's important to check with your doctor.

What's wrong with standing tall?

Nothing—unless you arch your back to do it.

It's estimated that 60 percent of America's working population have suffered from backaches at some time, and that employers and insurance companies spend billions of dollars paying for the treatment of those backs.

Ironically, many doctors believe that one significant cause of all that back trouble is the very posture so many of us are taught is "good": chest up, shoulders back, stomach flat, buttocks out. "Attention" posture—otherwise known as swayback.

One effect of swayback can be wear on the disks and aggravation of whatever disk problem may already affect your back. If, say, the disks already bulge and you stand arching your back, you might press those bulging disks onto neighboring nerves and cause yourself acute pain.

How can you tell about your posture? The American Medical Association in its *Book of Back Care* offers a very simple test. Lean against a wall or doorframe, touching it with both your upper back and buttocks. Slip your hand in the space between the wall and the small of your back. If your hand slips in easily, almost but not quite touching both the wall and your back, your posture's fine. If there's a big space between the wall and your back it means you're arching too much.

Here's an easy corrective exercise called pelvic tilt: Step a few inches from the wall. Try to flatten your entire back against it without bending your knees or hips. Tuck your tail under by rolling your pelvis up and under, tilting it.

Something else that might help you ease your back discomfort has its roots in the old saloons with footrails along the bar. Evidently putting a foot up on a rail made the back a lot more comfortable during imbibing. Doctors recommend the same for back sufferers, though not necessarily in a pub. Putting a foot on a low stool or a chair rung can bring relief from pain, because, among other reasons, it flattens out any spine arch and releases the tension on the sciatic nerve.

Whether you have good posture depends on your age, physique, health, even job. Generally speaking, you should stand so that each of your body's major sections—head, trunk, and legs—is balanced on the one below. This way gravity can't pull them out of alignment.

Are you likely to get postpartum blues?

Most women experience a brief letdown after having a baby. After all, their bodies have undergone enormous hormonal changes. And childbirth itself is much like running a big race: There's a lot of physical exertion, elation, and afterward a feeling of exhaustion and anticlimax. All of that is perfectly normal, and for most women the letdown feeling lasts about a week and then dissipates.

But some women—one in five, in fact—continue to feel depressed. They feel nervous and tired, always on the verge of tears. They can't eat, and they feel they can't cope, particularly with the new baby. Worst of all, they feel a lack of joy when they're with the new baby, and guilty as a result. After all, a mother isn't supposed to feel that way.

If this kind of depression lasts more than three weeks, it can be serious and should be treated immediately by professionals. Postpartum depression is like battle fatigue: The sooner it's treated, the sooner it's helped.

The causes are complex and vary from individual to individual. Part of it, of course, may be the drastic hormonal fluctuations that occur. Estrogen levels, which have risen about one hundred times during pregnancy, plummet to zero immediately after delivery. Similarly, the levels of progesterone, cortisol, thyroxine, and other hormones drop suddenly after childbirth, the lowest levels occurring about seventy-two hours after birth. Deficiencies in these hormones have been linked to depression. Recovery to normal levels usually occurs within a few weeks.

The psychological causes are even more complex, but there are some common threads. Experts have noted that postpartum depression can even be predicted in certain cases. Was the woman depressed before the baby arrived? Is the husband supportive? Are there excessive family worries about money, in-laws, marital problems? All these can be predicting factors. If they exist, it may be advisable to try to treat them before the baby comes. Talking out some of these problems in the presence of a trained therapist may help prevent more serious depression later on.

If you find yourself unable to shake off that blue feeling, don't hesitate to get help. There are now mothers' self-help groups, led by professionals, that offer mothers the support and encouragement they need. Or, if you prefer personal help, check your local mental-health center. It's comforting to know that help is available. Don't be ashamed to ask for it.

Whom do you call when you need advice about hiccups, or VD, or teething?

Ordinarily, the obvious answer is a doctor. But what if yours is out of town, or you are—or if you don't have a doctor at all? The answer then is a medical hotline—and it's free.

There are now a variety of telephone medical services, approved by medical societies and hospitals, that provide expert and confidential advice on almost all medical problems or emergencies. (These services are in addition to poison control centers, whose numbers are available in telephone directories for emergency situations involving the ingesting of poisonous materials.) The most ubiquitous of the services is TEL-MED, which was begun by the San Bernardino County (California) Medical Society and is now available in 320 communities in forty-six states. It plays on request a taped message, from three to six minutes long, on more than 350 subjects. If you think you might be pregnant, or your toddler's been bitten by a dog, or you suspect your teenager is taking drugs, or you're concerned about laxatives, diabetes, hypertension—whatever—TEL-MED has a tape in English or Spanish. If you can't find it listed in your telephone book, write to the TEL-MED office at P.O. Box 5249, San Bernardino, CA 92412, for the number nearest to your area.

Many other medical hotlines are staffed by either physicians or paraprofessionals who are prepared to listen and give direct assistance, especially for crisis intervention. Such facilities usually operate through hospitals or social-service agencies in large communities, and their phone numbers can be ascertained by calling a hospital or checking the phone book. For example, the Children's Hospital Medical Center in Boston offers pediatric advice by phone. Organizations also run hotlines. The American Digestive Disease Society sponsors Gutline, a service available on Tuesdays and Thursdays from 7:30 P.M. to 9 P.M. Eastern Time to answer questions about problems of the digestive system, from swallowing to diarrhea. Its number (in Maryland) is (301) 652-9293.

Hotline services have met with overwhelming approval from both consumers and physicians. In Pittsburgh alone, TEL-MED recently received a thousand requests for taped information in one day, and a survey reported satisfaction by 95 percent of its callers. Some valuable national numbers to have on hand include:

☐ Cancer Information Services, (800) 638-6694 (8 A.M. to midnight Eastern Time, seven days a week). Answers questions on all types of cancer, how to quit smoking, breast reconstruction, and the like.

☐ Women's Sports Foundation, (800) 227-3988 (9 A.M. to 5 P.M. Pacific Coast Time, weekdays); (415) 563-6266 (same times), California only. Sports medicine, pregnancy and running, fitness and health.

☐ Beech-Nut Infant Nutrition Hotline, (800) 523-6633 (9 A.M. to 4 P.M. Eastern Time, weekdays). Prenatal care, child development and nutrition.

☐ VD National Hotline, (800) 227-8922 (8 A.M. to 8 P.M. weekdays, or 8 A.M. to 6 P.M. weekends, Pacific Coast Time). Lists low-cost or no-fee referral services as well as providing answers to questions about the disease.

☐ Second Opinion Hotline, (800) 638-6833 (8 A.M. to midnight Eastern Time, seven days a week). Offers phone numbers of clinics and specialists for those who want a second opinion before deciding on surgery.

Why play safe on the ball field?

Because half of the nearly 1 million sports-related injuries youngsters suffer each year could have been prevented.

Here's what parents can do to help their children to injury-free athletic activities, according to pediatric-emergency experts:

☐ If you can have a say in the selection of a coach, pick one for more than athletic talent. The best coaches have degrees in physical education or health science, know first aid and cardiopulmonary resuscitation, and care more about kids having fun than about winning at any cost.

☐ Take your youngster for a complete physical exam, ideally by a physician who understands the specific demands of the sport the child wants to pursue.

☐ Make sure your child competes with a group of children of about the same size, weight, and degree of physical maturity. They will not necessarily all be the same age.

☐ Find out whether the playing field is safe. Inspect it for holes and obstacles. About 20 percent of sports injuries occur when children slam into such obstacles as parked cars and fences.

☐ Buy good equipment and see that your child uses it. This includes safety equipment. The American Dental Association recommends that children use mouth guards not just for contact sports like football, but for activities such as skateboarding as well. The American Academy of Ophthalmology points out that eye protectors or goggles can cut down on the more than four thousand eye injuries that occur each year during racket sports. (The best protector consists of a heavy-duty frame secured by a headband. A child who wears prescription glasses can have industrial-strength goggles ground to the prescription.) Feet sweat about one glass of water every day, and sneakers made of "nonbreathing" synthetic materials such as vinyl and nylon provide a perfect place for fungi and other microorganisms to breed. So see that your child uses canvas sneakers, ideally with a terry-cloth lining, and wash them frequently. Better yet, buy two pairs, and train your child to alternate wearing them. Buy cotton socks, which should, of course, be changed every day. Have the youngster use an antifungal powder as well.

☐ Insist that your youngster get into shape before beginning the sport, and stay in shape, too. Stretching exercises are particularly important; children often are not as limber as we think. Injuries are less frequent among children who are in good condition. An eight-year study published in the *American Journal of Sports Medicine* found that high-school football players who went through a preseason program of whole-body conditioning suffered fewer knee injuries than those who didn't, and the injuries they did get were less serious. The conditioning included cardiovascular stressing, acclimatization to heat, weight training, and exercises to improve flexibility and agility.

☐ Be aware of the risk in specific sports. About 20 percent of all children's sports injuries occur on the football field. In fact, most sports injuries occur in activities where collisions are likely, such as basketball, ice hockey, and roller skating. The injuries result not from the collision itself, but when the colliding youngsters hit the ground.

☐ If an injury does occur, make sure recovery is complete before you permit your child to resume play. Don't give in to pleas. And don't allow yourself to get so involved in your kid's athletic achievements that you push for a return to the field prematurely. Permanent damage could result.

When you've done what you can to make your child's athletic activity safe, relax. Bruises and cuts are likely to be the worst your youngster encounters; they account for about 80 percent of the sports injuries.

How can math multiply a girl's chances?

Just a basic knowledge of high-school algebra and geometry can add between $3,000 and $4,000 to a yearly paycheck. Yet many women are denied this extra earning power because they are victims of "math anxiety."

The anxiety can be defined as fear of figures. Its symptoms are the mind going blank, the girl's belief that she's "faking math" no matter how well she does in it, and feelings of helplessness, shame, and guilt in the face of what she sees as her failure at math. Many girls who suffer these symptoms give up math as soon as they can, in many cases early in high school.

A recent study of college freshmen by Lucy Sells, a sociologist at the University of Maryland, found that for every seven boys there was only one girl who had taken four years of high-school math—and that because of this 92 percent of the women students could not major in several popular fields of study, among them medicine, architecture, engineering, psychology, and science. For black freshmen in the study, the figures were even more bleak. Only 23 percent of the males and 10 percent of the females had four or more years of high-school math.

Why does math seem to be white-male territory? Experts believe that this is a cultural phenomenon, that historically women and black men have been directed toward low-level vocations requiring little or no mathematics.

According to Sheila Tobias, founder of the first math-anxiety clinic in the country, which was established at Wesleyan University, there are several reasons women have stayed away from math. One is the deep-seated fear that knowing math makes them unfeminine, or that they were born inadequate in math and their inferiority is "innate and irreversible." Tobias believes these feelings begin in early childhood with something so simple as the toys children are given. Boys customarily get playthings that help develop spatial and numerical skills; girls get toys that teach different skills.

The fears caused by math anxiety can be very costly. Aside from diminishing earning power, they deny sufferers the gratification of many interesting careers.

For those who are victims of math anxiety, there is help in the form of math clinics. Their premise is that the anxiety can be overcome through a combination of individual counseling, group work, experience sharing, even relaxation exercises and therapy sessions with a clinical psychologist if necessary. One such program, SummerMath at Mount Holyoke College in Massachusetts, has reported demonstrable success, turning anxiety-stricken young women, mostly juniors and seniors, into confident students able to program computers.

If you need help, check with a local school about the nearest clinics, or write to Catalyst, 14 East 60th Street, New York, NY 10022.

What's good for your cakes and your gums?

Baking soda and a pinch of salt. They can save you lots of dough.

Certain bacteria that commonly reside in our mouths often combine with food particles to form a hard plaque (calculus) between the teeth and gums. As the plaque builds up, it may cause pockets of inflammation to develop. If the condition is neglected, teeth begin to loosen as the gums recede, and the breath becomes acrid. To save the teeth, it is often necessary to undergo expensive and uncomfortable surgery to remove the plaque and treat the inflammation.

Ordinary brushing and flossing are not always enough to prevent this condition. Most Americans have gum disease, and it has been estimated that up to 75 percent of the cases begin in adolescence.

Is there an effective means of prevention? Some periodontists (dentists who specialize in gum disease) think that, in addition to brushing and flossing, a simple regimen involving baking soda, salt, and peroxide significantly lessens the accumulation of plaque. Researchers at the National Institutes of Health, who first reported the method, have verified the effectiveness of the ingredients as bacteria killers, at least in the test tube.

Here's how it works:

Put a small quantity of baking soda in a container and moisten with just enough hydrogen peroxide to form a thick paste. (Hydrogen peroxide is inexpensive and can be bought at a drugstore without prescription.) Smear the paste along the gums, front and back, and between the teeth. Using the rubber tip of a toothbrush, massage the gums and between the teeth. Then brush the teeth with a small toothbrush or an electric toothbrush. Next, irrigate the teeth and gums, especially in the areas where they meet, with a Water Pik filled with a mild salt solution. Run it at medium speed. In addition to its bactericidal properties, the salt helps shrink swollen gums, making it easier to get into the pockets. (People with high blood pressure can substitute Epsom salts for table salt.)

This treatment is still being evaluated, and there are periodontists who pooh-pooh it. But it's harmless and cheap. The one-time cost of the Water Pik is about $30.

How can you be seriously injured and not even know it?

Just by getting an earful of daily city living. And that doesn't include some of the super-loud music you hear these days. The trouble is, the ear can take a lot of punishment and damage without warning you through pain. It just doesn't complain out loud.

Hearing loss is an acute problem for the 20 million Americans the federal government says are subject to too much noise. But they and the rest of us can take steps to minimize the sounds of mayhem.

Most loud city and industrial sounds cause their damage gradually over long spells. Even modern conveniences such as electric razors, vacuum cleaners, food processors, and the like can, in time, seriously affect a person's hearing.

Hearing involves delicate mechanisms. The outer ear focuses sound vibrations into the eardrum, which vibrates and transfers the vibrations to tiny bones in the middle ear. These bones translate the sound vibrations into mechanical vibrations that are transmitted directly to the inner ear. Excessive sound does its damage to the inner-ear mechanism.

We measure sound in decibels, with zero being the point at which hearing begins. The decibel scale is logarithmic, meaning that every 10-decibel increase is perceived as being twice as loud. We hear normal breathing at 10 decibels. Normal conversation begins at 60 decibels, about twice as loud as the sound of moderate rainfall. Above that, says the Environmental Protection Agency, sound can be harmful to hearing.

A vacuum cleaner registers 75 decibels, heavy traffic 80, a power lawn mower 100, amplified rock music 120. The rock music, so pleasant to some ears, is twice as loud as a chain saw, sixteen times as loud as normal conversation. Dangerous? A test of a thousand college freshmen found that more than 60 percent had lost their hearing in the high-frequency range. That's why doctors and audiologists warn young people who wear Walkman sets or camp in their rooms with the volume up high on their stereos that they should turn the volume lower.

Adults who work in noisy places should wear soft-foam earplugs or even earmuffs to muffle industrial sounds around them. Rolling up the windows in the car keeps heavy traffic noises out.

As much as 50 percent of the noise level in your home can be cut. Radio and television might be kept in a room that is made sound-resistant with acoustical tiles and other insulation. Put rubber mats under appliances and use them only one at a time. Outside noises can be kept outside by weatherstripping windows and using solid or filled doors rather than hollow ones. Carpeting and drapes also help to absorb unwanted noise.

There are indications that sound hurts us in many ways other than physical. Studies have shown that chronic exposure to heightened sound levels raises the blood pressure, induces or irritates ulcers, and produces fatigue and irritability. In school-children it reduces concentration and the ability to perform well on tests. Even the fetus in the womb is not totally immune to outside noise.

So pay attention to the noise around you. Tune it down or one of these days, when it is quiet enough to hear a pin drop, you won't be able to.

What's one reason students drop out of college?

Some of them experience anxiety, depression, and even panic. Some have physical symptoms such as nausea, headaches, sleeplessness, and loss of appetite. Some can't concentrate. Some feel tightness in their heads or chests, muscle cramps, and even a sense of impending doom. Yet all of these symptoms, from the mild to the terrifying, can be traceable to an emotion we usually attribute to children much younger than college age: homesickness. Especially in their freshman year, they just can't adjust to their new environment and yearn passionately to return to familiar people and places. The result: A substantial number, mostly young women, drop out of college.

Students are embarrassed to admit they're homesick, so the cause may not be obvious to a concerned adult. They equate homesickness with immaturity, and don't want to discuss it. College life is supposed to be exciting and desirable, and they're reluctant to admit that they're having trouble adjusting.

Parents can ease a child's transition from home to college, counselors advise, by discussing the possibility of homesickness before the child departs for school. Students should understand that it's a normal, common feeling, that being homesick doesn't mean there's something wrong with them, or with the college.

Students who do develop homesickness can drive it away by flinging themselves into an active college life. In addition to academic activities, they should attend sporting events, and take advantage of the cultural life as well as the social life at the college. They should work hard at making new friends—for example, by joining church groups and clubs. Feelings of loss and isolation ordinarily vanish quickly as new students become more involved in collegiate life.

Students who find their homesickness lingers or is very intense should drop by a college counseling center right away. Almost all colleges have them nowadays. Their staffs are trained to help homesick students—and to discourage them from dropping out before they've really given themselves a chance to succeed.

Do you resent your eight-month-old baby?

If you do, don't feel guilty. The "baby honeymoon" of the first few months is over, and it's time to take a realistic look at the changes that parenthood has made in your life.

According to a recent study by Dr. Brent C. Miller and Donna L. Sollie, the typical parent experiences a slight decline in morale as well as an increase in marital and personal stress toward the end of the first year of parenthood. New mothers experience these feelings more than new fathers. For both parents, however, the new baby has meant lack of sleep, tiredness, increased work around the house, and feelings of overwhelming responsibility and being tied down. The baby has also meant that parents have had less time for themselves and each other. Frequently, wives begin complaining that their husbands are not paying enough attention to them. The couple's social and recreational life has been severely disrupted, and they've had little time to spend with their friends. Their life, once predictable and orderly, is now somewhat chaotic.

Coping with these normal stresses of parenthood involves learning, patience, and the ability to become more flexible. It's important to maintain a sense of continuity and to realize that the situation will get better as time goes on. Seeking out friends and neighbors for advice helps, but hiring a baby-sitter while you take a refreshing break may be just what you need to get back on the track.

Parenthood consists of good times and bad times. A new baby can give added meaning to life and strengthen the bond between you and your spouse. Realizing that parenthood has both positive and negative aspects and being honest about your feelings—including feelings of resentment—will result in your truly enjoying your baby even more.

What drink is best for the summer athlete?

Water. Whether for the summer athlete or anyone else caught in summer's heat, the most refreshing and most restorative liquid you can drink is a cold glass of good old reliable H_2O.

Unless you're acclimated to warm weather and in top physical condition, strenuous exercise is risky in hot weather. If you plan to exercise, do it in the early morning or in the evening, when the sun is down, and take ten minutes of rest for every hour of exercise. Also, drink a glass of water half an hour beforehand, and while exercising stop every ten or fifteen minutes to drink water. Afterward drink another glass of water every twenty minutes for about two hours, even if you don't feel thirsty.

The idea is to avoid dehydration, which can cause heat exhaustion or, worse, heatstroke—and that kills more than five hundred people every summer. Victims of heat exhaustion get cold and clammy, perspire profusely, and often get cramps in their leg and abdominal muscles. If you start to feel that way, get into a cool, shady place immediately and lie down with your head lower than your body. Pressure with a wet, warm towel should help the cramps. Drink a mild salty liquid.

Heatstroke, caused when the body can't eliminate its excess heat, is more serious and requires more drastic treatment. Symptoms are a rapid pulse, a temperature of 106° F or higher, and sometimes red, hot skin. Victims are also often disoriented, if not unconscious, and should be taken to a doctor or hospital immediately. If an ambulance has to be summoned, the victim should be wrapped in a cold wet sheet while waiting for it. Try cooling the body by sponging with alcohol or warm water.

By the way, stay away from soft drinks when exercising, because they're not as good for you as water, and to be effective they have to be diluted with water, some in a ratio of as much as seven to one. Caffeine drinks will speed metabolism, so avoid colas and coffee and tea, even if iced.

Does a mastectomy have to be radical?

For nearly a century a diagnosis of breast cancer routinely led to a radical mastectomy, in which surgeons removed the entire breast as well as lymph nodes in the armpit and chest muscle tissue. It was the best, in fact only, treatment available. But today doctors are studying less drastic surgery.

An eight-year study at the National Cancer Institute in Milan, Italy, of 701 patients with early breast cancer—defined as tumors less than three quarters of an inch in diameter—compared radical mastectomy with removal of only the quadrant of the breast containing the malignancy. It found that the more extensive surgery was "unnecessary mutilation." In this study women fared equally well with only the "quadrantectomy," followed by several weeks of radiation therapy.

In the future, doctors may be able to offer women an even more minimal operation, lumpectomy, in which only the malignancy and a little of the surrounding tissue is cut away. The effectiveness of this approach is being appraised, too.

Recently, doctors from the Division of Plastic Surgery of the Medical College of Virginia reported that "modified" radical mastectomy—in which the nerve supply to the pectoralis major muscle was preserved—facilitated breast reconstruction after surgery. They said there was no evidence that the reconstruction enhanced recurrence of the cancer.

The key to saving the breast is catching the cancer early, and researchers are exploring paths to this goal. At the University of Wisconsin Hospital in Madison, doctors are using refined computerized ultrasound scanning to detect tumors less than a quarter of an inch in diameter. Elsewhere researchers are trying to develop a special brassiere that contains sensors to pick up hot spots in breast tissue that could signal a malignancy. Still, today, aside from mammography, the best screening tool is your own hands, used in a monthly self-examination of your breasts. Ask your doctor or local cancer society for information on how to do it.

―――――――――――――――

What's the best cure for a broken heart?

Time. It may or may not heal all wounds, but for a broken heart it's the right prescription.

Falling in love again soon, on the other hand, won't heal the heart. On the contrary, it might just get in the way of the mending process.

Recent studies show that at the end of a love relationship your body actually suffers physical deprivation. It turns out the "chemistry" of love is real. It's called phenylethylamine, and it creates a response somewhat like an amphetamine high. When a love affair ends, the brain of the spurned lover stops producing the phenylethylamine and immediately starts feeling its loss. The resulting symptoms are very much like those of amphetamine withdrawal, primarily depression and apathy. (If you find yourself gorging on chocolate, you might be trying to cure yourself; chocolate is full of phenylethylamine.)

Most broken hearts heal themselves in six months to a year. The anger, frustration, and hostility that follow an ended relationship will fade in time. Doing things with friends, trying new and different kinds of activities that will bring new people into your life, casual dating, maybe joining a group of people who are going through the same pain and can share their experiences—all these activities help the cure. But rushing headlong into another serious relationship before you're healed will most likely bring you more pain. In order to enjoy a successful love you have to come to terms with the one that's past. You have to understand yourself and others. If you take enough time to do that and to let your broken heart mend, you'll be ready to try again, and this time you'll have a better sense of what you're doing.

For some people, however, the pain of a broken heart does not heal with time. Their suffering is prolonged and serious, and they are unable to cope, unsure of themselves, moody, often unable to function at work. So if time does not mend a broken heart, consider help from a therapist.

What's music to your ailments?

Whether a dose of Beethoven or the Beatles, music can be medicinal.

Recent research has shown music to be effective therapy for ailments ranging from drug addiction to headaches. Increasingly, dentists are using it to relax patients and to distract them from the sound of the drill. At the Royal Victoria Hospital in Montreal, classical music is so effective a painkiller for cancer patients that many have been taken off analgesic drugs. Doctors at the University of Kansas Medical Center in Kansas City discovered that music in the delivery room shortens labor and cuts down on the need for anesthesia. And doctors in another midwestern hospital found that music eases the anxieties of preoperative patients, makes administering anesthesia easier, and decreases the incidence of postoperative vomiting.

In Poland, research shows music to be an effective antidote to headaches and neurological diseases. Of 408 people studied over a six-month period, half listened to symphonic music, the other half to no music at all. After the six months the music listeners were using fewer sedatives and painkillers.

Doctors cannot yet explain why music is proving such an effective therapy. Dr. Leo Shatin, president of the American Association for Music Therapy, thinks one reason is the human inability to respond fully to simultaneous stimuli. If music becomes the dominant stimulus, it displaces others. Other doctors point out that the more you like a piece of music the more deeply you breathe when you listen to it, and consequently the more you relax.

Whatever the reason for it, to use music to relax or change mood, three basic musical elements—pitch, volume, and tempo—are involved.

Pitch is quite simply the number of vibrations a sound wave produces. Something in a high pitch has more waves and creates tension. Something pitched low, with fewer vibrations per second, will be relaxing.

Volume, if it's high enough, can actually cause pain and serious damage to the ear. The average rock concert is ninety decibels, which is a harmful level, but some people wrap themselves in loud music as a way of protecting themselves, of relieving, at least temporarily, their feelings of insecurity.

From the time we hear our mother's heartbeat in the uterus, tempo affects us profoundly. If it's much faster than the heartbeat (seventy to eighty beats a minute), tempo can make us tense or excited. If it's slower, it can create suspense. If it's approximately the same as the heartbeat, it can relax us. If its rhythm is different from that of the heart, it can affect us as well, sometimes profoundly. Dr. John Diamond, president of the International Academy of Preventive Medicine, says there is certain rock music that can cause a temporary loss of as much as two thirds of a body's muscular strength. Its beat is anapestic (two short beats followed by one loud, long one—di di DAH), which is exactly opposite the heart's rhythm (DAH di di). The Rolling Stones' music is anapestic, the Beatles' isn't. How you want to feel will determine which one you want to play, but neither will be as therapeutic as Frank Sinatra or folk music. And Beethoven, according to Dr. Diamond, is more therapeutic than any of them.

If you want to use music to change your mood, start with the kind that fits the way you're feeling and then select what leads your mood progressively to where you want it to be. Whatever you choose—fast, loud music to excite you or quiet, cheerful music of a moderate beat to relax by—if you play the same music all day long it can irritate, even tire you. So, Doctor, what's the recommended dosage? According to Dr. Shatin, take your music in twenty- to forty-minute doses, a few times a day.

Do myths about menstruation still prevail?

Alas, they do. And most of them are just as wrong and as damaging to women as they always have been. Fortunately, there's been a great deal of research into menstruation in recent years, and the myths can be dispelled.

One is that menstrual cramps are psychological. They're not. About 60 percent of menstruating women experience dysmenorrhea (the Greek word for painful menstrual flow). For most of them the pain, fortunately, is mild. But as many as 14 percent of American teenage girls go through such pain that they frequently stay home and miss school. And while the common pattern of dysmenorrhea is that it tapers off as a woman gets older, for many women it continues, intensely in some cases, until menopause. But it is *not* mental. Recent research has placed the pain where it originates—in the uterus—and has shown that it is definitely biological.

Experts now think that a major cause of menstrual cramps is the increase of a substance in the uterine lining called prostaglandin. It stimulates the muscles of the uterus. The resulting pain, which can begin two days or so before the actual flow, intensifies on the first day of menstruation and can last anywhere from a few hours to two days.

Good news, though: There are remedies—of all sorts. Heat, applied to either the lower back or the abdominal area, can help; so can a well-conditioned body, a well-balanced diet, and, for many women, a drink or two. Alcohol seems to relax the muscles in the uterine wall. You can also try acupressure: Rub the area an inch to the right of your spine at your midback. The pain should subside in thirty or forty seconds, disappear in three or four minutes, and not return for up to six hours.

If none of this helps, there is medicine. Doctors have long known that the use of oral contraceptives can help in reducing menstrual pain, but for those who eschew them there is aspirin, as well as some newer prescription drugs called antiprostaglandins.

The secret is to prevent the prostaglandin from producing uterine cramps, so it's important to take the drugs *before* the cramp starts.

Similarly, premenstrual syndrome, called by the *Journal of the American Medical Association* "an ancient woe deserving of modern scrutiny," can be treated now. For some women the symptoms—breast tenderness, bloating, irritability, and depression—are so intense that they can be relieved only with hormones. But other women can take care of the symptoms themselves. How? First, find out whether you suffer from the syndrome. Keep a calendar of your menstrual days and your moods. If, after three months, you detect a pattern around your period, you probably have PMS. You can then experiment by cutting down on salt to help with water retention and boosting your potassium and vitamin B_6 intake; both of them may affect your mood. Eat small but frequent meals, and if you have cravings, indulge them before your period. This way you can help keep up your blood-sugar level, which tends to fall premenstrually. If none of this helps you, see your doctor.

Let's not forget that age-old myth that menstruating women are less physically and intellectually competent. It's not true. Menstruating women competing in Olympics have won bronze, silver, and gold medals. In fact, one American woman won three gold medals and broke a world's record at the height of her period.

As for intellectual deterioration during menstruation, studies at Princeton and Yale show that if it occurs it does so because the woman to whom it happens was conditioned to expect it. In fact, the Yale study concluded that women actually did better on tests when they were menstruating; rather than have to cope with an undefined anxiety, they could pinpoint the source of their distress, deal with it, and then think more clearly.

If women—and men—sweep away the musty myths and look at menstruation with an informed and rational eye, they could think more clearly, too.

Guess who's looking for a roommate?

The senior citizen who doesn't want or can't afford to live alone. A growing number are trying a new option—shared housing. It's an alternative that can save between 50 and 75 percent of their housing costs, and makes it possible for the elderly to feel secure, pay their bills, and enjoy companionship.

There are scores of shared-housing projects scattered around the country: communes in Baltimore, a townhouse in Boston, group housing in California, to name a few. The number of participants ranges from the 3 sharing an apartment in Brookline, Massachusetts, to 125 in "Share a Home" in Winter Park, Florida.

Whatever the size of the project, members usually have at least one private room, and in some cases a private bathroom, too. They share common living rooms, dining rooms, kitchens, and laundry facilities. Their rents are prorated, and they usually include utilities and basic phone costs.

Although almost all shared-housing projects have full-time or part-time staff and administrative help, members often share food shopping, cooking, and other chores. Most households hold regularly scheduled meetings so that all members can participate in decisions necessary to keep the household running harmoniously. They can also hire—and fire—the staff, and vote on the admission of new members.

Shared-housing projects are usually located in a large, existing house in a stable neighborhood, because, for one thing, renovating an old house is less expensive than building a new one.

There are, however, drawbacks for the very poor. Some government subsidies such as welfare benefits may be reduced when a person joins a shared-housing unit.

For free brochures on existing projects and on starting your own, write Shared Housing Resource Center, 6344 Greene Street, Philadelphia, PA 19144. You might discover that you're never too old to share.

How can time cause a skin rash?

The back of your wristwatch may contain nickel. This metal, widely used in making watches, earrings, rings, and bracelets, is one of the most common causes of skin rashes. About one in every ten people wearing such jewelry eventually gets an allergic reaction.

There is an amazing array of other substances and materials that can cause rashes in sensitive people. In fact, almost any substance coming into contact with the skin may cause reactions in some people.

A study by dermatologists in ten major medical centers has

come up with a list of the most common causes of skin rashes. These include, besides nickel, potassium dichromate, commonly found in tanned leather and watchbands; antiseptics containing thimerosal or merthiolate; and the ingredient p-phenylenediamine, used in hair dyes.

A skin rash can also be caused by perfume, which may consist of sixty or more components, including natural products and extracts from flowers, plants, roots, herbs, gums, and animals, as well as aromatic chemicals. Numerous medicines can incite rashes, too; for example, some women develop skin outbreaks from using vaginal medications. So varied, so individual, and so widespread are skin reactions that the Food and Drug Administration has set up a National Registry of Dermatological Reactions to Drugs to enable dermatologists to report cases anytime, around the clock.

If you get a puzzling skin rash, try to get at the cause by eliminating one possible suspect after another in things you use, wear, or eat. If that doesn't work, check with your doctor.

Do I have a right to see my child's school records?

Absolutely, no matter what grade the child is in. And so does your child, if the records in question are those of the Scholastic Aptitude Tests (SATs).

The federal Family Education Rights and Privacy Act gives parents the right to inspect, challenge, and insert corrections into children's school records. Because those records can affect your children's future education and career, you may want to make it your business to know what's in them.

Records frequently contain false or damaging information and schools have been known to release records to people who have no right to them. For example, a woman in Texas discovered that her child's records contained an unfounded accusation that the youngster was a kleptomaniac. Another parent was told by a guidance counselor who was preparing a college application that the youth had been labeled a "possible schizophrenic" back in elementary school.

As for high-school students, they are in a better position to profit from the past than they used to be, because they now have access to their SATs—not just the test scores, but copies of the questions, the correct answers, and their own answers. Answers for the PSATs, the "practice" SATs usually taken by high-school juniors, are also available. The service costs $6.50. Students can place orders anytime after they receive admission tickets to the SATs, up to five months after the test date. For information, write College Board Admissions Testing Program, Box 592-D, Princeton, NJ 08541.

Just about every kind of school record is covered by the federal law except an individual teacher's personal notes not kept in the master file. The law specifies grades, IQ scores, results of psychological tests, notes on behavior, reports by counselors, and the results of tests for the handicapped.

You can ask to see the records by writing to the principal of your child's school. The school must respond within forty-five days.

If you disagree with something you find in a record, you can ask the school to change it. If the school refuses, the law provides for an impartial hearing, and for legal advice to your family. The officer in charge of the hearing will have no connection with the school system and can order the records changed. Even if the hearing officer decides not to issue such an order, you can still insist that a statement opposing the disputed information be put in your child's file.

For more information, write Family Education Rights and Privacy Act, Department of Education, Room 4512, Switzer Building, Washington, DC 20202.

━━━━━━━━━━━━━━━━━

What's blue about the flu?

The answer could be you and something known as post-influenza depression. Called the wobblies, the blues, or the blahs, they go on for a time after a bout with influenza and its chills, fever, nausea, aches, and bad dreams.

The problem is most people don't realize that it's the aftermath of the flu and think something may be seriously wrong with them.

Look at it this way. A virus attacks your body—and some strains are pretty vicious. All your body's immune defenses are mobilized. Your major organs may spring to the defense—the lungs, liver, lymph system, intestinal tract. No wonder you feel exhausted, weak, and depressed after the battle is won.

What it means is that you should take more time to recover. Be sure to get lots of sleep and rest, and eat a sensible diet, with lots of liquids. Don't rush back to work before you feel really back to normal. By the way, the same kind of fatigue, mental and physical, often follows other viral infections such as mononucleosis, the so-called kissing disease, and hepatitis, the liver infection.

Don't worry, a case of the flu won't cause you to go bananas. Two Irish researchers, Drs. Kenneth Sinanan and Irene B. Hillary, writing in the *British Journal of Psychiatry* about a study they did, say they found no relationship between a flu attack and clinical depression that was severe enough to require the help of a psychiatrist.

Depression following the flu is temporary. You most likely can and will lick it on your own.

What can cause both buzzing in your head and ringing in your ears?

Your jaw. Specifically, tense jaw. Besides migraines and tinnitus, it can cause excruciating face pain or earache, bring on lopsided faces and deformed lips, and produce dizziness. And it's made worse by bad habits such as clenching the teeth during the day or grinding the teeth when you're asleep, things many people do.

The troubles all can stem from the temporomandibular joint, where, near the ears, the lower jaw or mandible meets the temporal bone of the skull. This is the hinge of the jaw. The two bony parts are separated by a small disk, but they essentially operate as a ball-and-socket joint, held together by ligaments. Powerful jaw muscles permit movement up and down, and also sideways to some extent, as you can tell by moving your jaw.

But things can, and do, go wrong with such an arrangement, and some 20 million Americans develop jaw problems bringing on a raft of symptoms, classified as the TMJ syndrome. Women are four times more likely to develop TMJ than men.

A major cause of TMJ is malocclusion, meaning your teeth don't come together correctly. One high filling can throw the alignment off, or malocclusion may result from a missing tooth, or damage to the jaw. Dentists have well-practiced skills to correct such causes, and can use a bite plate to retrain jaw muscles and to reduce grinding of the teeth.

TMJ may be a psychosomatic problem as well, says Dr. Walter Guralnick, professor of oral and maxillofacial surgery at the Harvard School of Dental Medicine. He says that in many cases the jaw can be relaxed with hot packs, muscle relaxants, and pain relievers. He also recommends a soft diet to reduce chewing, and retraining of the jaw muscles. Biofeedback techniques might help some people with this condition.

And there's a simple exercise called the quieting reflex that anyone can perform for a few minutes at a time to reduce jaw-muscle tension. Let your jaw hang open, moving it back and forth to a pain-free position. Gently massage the jaw muscles; then close your eyes and relax, staying that way for a minute.

What does your garbage say?

That you're probably throwing away money.

In the mid-1970s a group of researchers at the University of Arizona collected data on household refuse in the city of Tucson. What they discovered down in the dumps was that the average family was discarding about $100 or more of edible food a year. Put in national terms, that would come to $4.5 billion worth, or enough to feed 20 million people. And what the researchers found did not include what they couldn't see—the food that went down the drain, onto the compost heap, or into the dog's dish.

According to Professor William Rathje, one of the research group, "knowledge is one of the most important elements in food waste, knowledge of when food is and isn't safe to eat. We found that families that knew the answers discarded around 25 percent less edible food than those who didn't."

Many people, fearful of food poisoning, follow the principle "When in doubt throw it out." Others unwittingly jeopardize their health, or the health of others, by keeping foods too long.

Spoilage is caused by bacterial contamination. Some foods

are more hospitable hosts to bacteria than others. Bacteria will not multiply at freezer temperatures. However, if in thawing, the food or outer portion of the food is allowed to reach the 45°–140° range for any length of time, the bacteria will multiply to the point of dangerous contamination.

So be sure that your freezer is never above zero degrees Fahrenheit. Equally important, wrap all your freezer foods in moisture-proof paper, bags, foil, or containers.

It's also essential to realize that freezing is not forever; that even if wholesomeness is not affected, enzymes and oxidation may cause loss of quality in nutrition, color, texture, and flavor. Foods such as ham, bacon, and sausage can be safely stored in the freezer for two months; ice cream and sherbet for one month; whole chicken or turkey, a year; fish, six months (unless it's fatty fish, which lasts only three months); broths, gravy, potato salad, and cooked organ meats not at all—eat them in a couple of days. (See Appendix A for additional storage information.) One lesson to be learned from even this partial list is that buying in bulk may not always be a bargain.

Fortunately, you don't have to be a graduate nutritionist to be food and dollar-wise. The Department of Agriculture now has a central consumer service from which you can get answers to questions regarding the cooking, storing, and quality of meat and poultry. Write to Food and Safety Consumer Inquiries, Room 1163-S, Department of Agriculture, Washington, DC 20250, or call (202) 472-4485. The service will also send publications on request.

Why do babies, of all people, prefer peace and quiet?

Because they have to study. Babies begin learning almost from the moment they are born, and parents have long been encouraged to provide environmental stimulation to aid the process. But contrary to Mae West's well-known assertion that "too much of a good thing is wonderful," too much stimulation, too many competing noises, can stymie the process. In fact, says Theodore D. Wachs, a psychologist at Purdue University, too much may be as bad as too little.

Unlike older siblings, who are seemingly able to absorb simultaneously plane geometry and the sounds of the latest Grateful Dead album, babies and small children need to focus their concentration. Noise may interfere with a baby's ability to discriminate between stimuli. Dr. Wachs's research shows that a high level of household noise—from radios, record players, appliances, people, and especially television, going all the time—is related to inhibited intellectual development.

Seven-month-old infants observed in homes where they were exposed to excessive noise showed below-average development in imitating gestures and in their ability to manipulate objects. Eighteen-month-olds were deficient in their comprehension of space and early memory. Infants who at six months had been exposed to too much distraction and relentless noise at twenty-four months showed significant delays in the development of language skills. They were also delayed in initiating exploratory behavior, an indication that the blossoming of normal curiosity had been thwarted.

Not surprisingly, male babies proved much more sensitive in this regard than female babies, tending to reinforce the view that males are intrinsically more vulnerable to stress. Temperamental differences also played a role: Easygoing, placid babies were less adversely affected than high-strung, difficult ones.

So concentrate your baby's attention. Don't overwhelm it. Music, the vacuum cleaner, your voice, a rattle, a singing commercial on the TV—they're all sounds for baby to study and to learn from, but not all at once and not all the time.

When is the school lunch box a hotbed of disease?

When bacteria are allowed to fester in it for two hours or more. The result can be food poisoning. So if your child comes home from school complaining of dizziness, abdominal cramps, diarrhea, or vomiting—or all of these symptoms—don't pass it off as a touch of the flu. It might be food poisoning, and it might happen again unless you change the way you make lunch and pack it.

Because food poisoning is often mistaken for flu and because it is seldom reported, experts think that it is far more widespread than is commonly believed. Only rarely are any kinds of food poisoning fatal. Botulism is an exception, but it is extremely rare:

In 89 percent of the known botulism cases over the last eight years the cause has been home-canned foods that were not processed correctly. Most other kinds of food poisoning are over within thirty-six hours, although some strains can last as long as a week and can recur.

The most common causes of food poisoning are meats and dairy products that have been improperly prepared or stored. To avoid it, keep hot foods hot, cold foods cold, and all foods clean. Bacteria thrive at temperatures between 45° and 140° F. At temperatures below or above that, most are harmless.

This means that you want to exercise climate control in your child's lunch box. The best way is to buy a vacuum bottle to use for either hot or cold liquids. A commercial freezer-gel pack will keep your solids chilled, as will lidded plastic containers filled with ice and then frozen. You can also, if you apply sauces or condiments sparingly, freeze meat sandwiches the night before. Then, when you pack them, they will keep other foods chilled and will defrost in time for lunch. Be prepared, though, for a loss in quality.

Whatever you serve for lunch, make sure that it's clean, that you prepare it in a clean place with clean implements, and that you pack it in a clean box or bag. Wash off your utensils and countertops with soap and water. If you use a lunch box, wash it with soap and water after every use. Vacuum bottles should be cleaned with boiling water. And if you brown-bag it, be sure to use a clean, previously unused bag each day. If you include fresh fruits and vegetables, scrub them, too.

If your child's school has a lunch program, it may be worth considering it. A recent U.S. Department of Agriculture study of seven thousand families throughout the United States found that students participating in school lunch programs were doing better nutritionally than students who were not.

Related studies conducted in several states also show that the nutrition in school lunches costs less than in lunch-box meals. For example, in Fairfax, Virginia, a lunch consisting of a turkey sandwich on a roll, carrot and celery sticks, and fresh fruit cost $1.05 if prepared at home; 75 cents for elementary students and 85 cents for secondary-school students if purchased in school.

Most school lunches offer several choices and, according to the Department of Agriculture, are demonstrably more sanitary than lunches carried from home. They could take the work and worry out of at least one of the day's meals.

Is sex always crucial in a marriage?

Not all the time. If it were, there would be even more divorces than there are.

A flood of marital guides and popular articles seem to suggest that sex is the be-all and end-all of a successful marriage. But according to studies of married men and women, sex is sometimes far less important than other factors.

The Department of Psychiatry of the University of Pittsburgh School of Medicine conducted a study of one hundred couples who considered their marriages successful. Over 90 percent said that if they had to do it over, they would marry the same person, and 80 percent viewed their sexual relations as satisfying. Yet "satisfying" obviously took in a lot of territory, because more than half the women and four in ten men reported serious sexual dysfunction. And nearly a third of the couples had sexual intercourse only two or three times a month or less—far below average. As the researchers observed, "It is not the quality of sexual performance but the affective tone of the marriage that determines how most couples perceive the quality of their sexual relations."

Sol Gordon, a psychologist who directs the Institute for Family Research and Education at Syracuse University and has studied hundreds of marriages, places sex behind trust, loyalty, laughter, tolerance, and adaptability as a factor in keeping marriages happy and working. Love, he says, "means more than romance and passion. It means really liking each other and being friends."

Marriage, like friendship, involves having understanding and compassion not only for the other person's needs but for one's own as well, and being willing to communicate them openly. Partners who are afraid to express anger or who hide their feelings for fear of rejection can build a wall of rage and hostility between them. They may think certain feelings are "wrong." For example, we are told that separate beds discourage sexuality and intimacy. But it's hard to feel loving when you're kept awake at night by a snoring or thrashing partner. Better a special close time and then a separate, but equal, night's sleep.

Another myth is that men resist marriage. The time is past when marriage was the only assurance a man had of an available sex partner, yet the vast majority of men continue to marry. According to a report in the journal *Medical Aspects of Human Sexuality*, 96 percent of American men have married or plan to, and a representative sampling said that the most important quality they seek in a wife is someone to be "totally honest and open with." Only one in four mentioned sexual excitement.

On the other hand, sex *is* an important part of human life and pleasure. A partner who feels that his or her sexual relationship is less than it should be need not feel constrained about questioning a spouse's attitudes. Help through counseling and therapy is available and often effective.

What, indeed, is in a name?

Future success, if you believe the experts.

Psychologists and onomatologists (name scholars) tell us that what we name our children can dramatically affect the rest of their lives. Children with common names, such as Robert, Michael, Sally, or Jennifer, tend to be more popular and to do better in school than children with so-called undesirable names, according to a number of studies, including that of Harvard psychologist Robert Rosenthal.

These studies also show that a child's self-confidence can be directly affected by his or her name. As early as kindergarten, it influences a child's ability to adjust. Children react to their own and others' names, and several studies show that how much people like their own name bears directly on how well adjusted they are. Children with nicknames, for example, tend to be better adjusted; they see the nickname as a sign of affection.

Whether we like it or not, certain names carry personality stereotypes, and very often children with those names will assume varying degrees of those stereotypes. Bertha is often thought of as a "fat" name, Percy as "weak," Gertrude as "ugly," Milton as "passive." On the other hand, Katie is "spirited," Jean is "straightforward," Bill is "dependable," John is "stolid." Moreover, according to studies, a "Jr." scores lower than a man with Roman numerals after his name on traits such as tolerance, well-being, and responsibility.

One study—which included a class of Harvard graduates, child patients of a New Jersey psychiatric institution, and mental patients in a Chicago institution—indicated that people with "odd" or outlandish first names such as Throckmorton and Precious more frequently had behavior problems. And Loyola University psychologists found that people with "peculiar" first names (Lethal and Vere being two mentioned) committed four times the number of criminal acts as people whose names were more ordinary.

Of course, this can cut two ways. Some people feel their unusual name makes them special. After all, amidst the Georges, Thomases, and Jameses who were President, there were Millard, Calvin, Ulysses, Grover, and Woodrow.

Today a variety of names are flourishing, from Victorian ones such as Emma and Amanda to idiosyncratic, biblical, and ethnic names. Experts advise expectant parents to think about a number of factors before naming their child:

- [ ] Consider the effect of the name on the child.
- [ ] Choose one that is not sexually ambiguous.
- [ ] Be able to spell and pronounce the name without difficulty.
- [ ] And think about what nickname might be made of the name, or initials, whether it rhymes with anything embarrassing, or whether a name that's cute at age two—like Peanuts or Little Boo—will be ludicrous at age twenty.

Does it make sense to talk to your baby?

Absolutely—the more conversation the better. Oral communication skills are vital in themselves, and also the foundation for learning to read. Study after study has shown that children who have learned to carry on an interesting conversation with their parents do better in school.

Even before a baby first mutters, "Dada," parents should repeat the baby's babbling sounds. The baby thus realizes the parents are pleased, and is encouraged to try again. Research indicates that babies who are talked to and stimulated by speech speak better and talk earlier. But "baby talk" at the "dada" stage should not be encouraged.

In order to learn how to speak, children need lots of experience with actual words and language. They should hear all kinds of words and word patterns. Even though babies don't understand, they love the sounds of language, especially the musical sounds of nursery rhymes and jingles. Repeat these over and over again to your baby.

As your infant gets older and really begins to converse, keep the child talking. Keep it natural, though, and make sure your interest is real. Kids can spot a phony, and they'll lose interest. Ask real questions and pursue them. "What did you like about it?" "Why?" "Did it make you feel happy or sad?" Listen carefully to your child's response, and don't talk down.

Reading aloud to your child is one of the best methods of stimulating conversation and is vital for the child's learning to read. Read your child's favorite stories over and over again, and let the child see the book as you read. Children learn the structure of the language—and the appearance of words on a page—by going over and over the same story. Research indicates that seeing the words as they are read is important in developing prereading and beginning reading skills.

Point-and-say books are particularly helpful. While reading out loud, point to an illustration, name it, and talk about it. "See the dog." After a while, the child will learn to point to the dog, and a conversation can begin. "What color is the dog?" "Is the dog big?" "Does the dog have a tail?"

By the time a child is five, he or she knows about two thousand words and can understand the basic sentence structure of language in a remarkably sophisticated way. This is the time to encourage reading on his or her own.

The quarterback—should he or shouldn't he the night before a game?

Terry Bradshaw and Fran Tarkenton might have something to say about that question. In the 1975 Super Bowl, Bradshaw was the quarterback for the Pittsburgh Steelers, who were allowed to spend the night before the game with their wives. Tarkenton quarterbacked the Minnesota Vikings; they were isolated from their wives. The Steelers won, 16–6.

Speaking strictly physically, sexual intercourse before a big game—or, for that matter, before a track meet, boxing match, or tennis match—won't hurt an athlete's performance.

The old myth that sexual activity will sap an athlete's strength is just that—an old myth. The average man uses only four to six calories a minute during intercourse. That's roughly what he'd use to take a quick walk around the block.

According to Dr. Donald L. Cooper, director of Oklahoma State University's Hospital and Clinic in Stillwater and team physician for the Big Eight Conference representatives, athletes who are married or who have regular sexual partners can be relaxed by pregame sex. It might even help them sleep better. So it's not surprising that many medical experts believe that sex the night before a contest will have no effect on the performance of athletes if sexual intercourse is a regular part of their lives.

Now here's a turnabout question: What will engaging in *athletics before sex* do to sexual performance?

If tests by Dr. J. R. Sutton of the Garvan Institute of Medicine in Australia are an indication, exercise improves sex. He measured the testosterone levels of athletes and nonathletes before, during, and after vigorous exercise. The levels were highest after exercise, and they were higher in the athletes than in the nonathletes. There are two possible explanations for this: that exercise improves blood circulation, which in turn generates healthy distribution of testosterone, the hormone believed responsible for the male sex drive; or that testosterone helps the muscles store their favorite fuel, glycogen, so the more the muscles are used the more testosterone will be produced.

Exercise, it seems, is a natural aphrodisiac.

When is saving money hazardous to your health?

When you turn your home thermostat down too low—65° or below. The danger is hypothermia, meaning that your body temperature falls to 95 degrees Fahrenheit or less (98.6, of course, is normal). Hypothermia can creep up on us, on elderly people particularly.

The gradual loss in body temperature slows down the heartbeat and metabolism, the pulse grows weaker, and less nourishing blood flows to the brain. A person then becomes less alert, less likely to realize he or she is really becoming cold, and less likely to do something about it. The situation happens frequently to skiers and climbers who suddenly find themselves chilled and sweating after a day on the mountains.

Accidental hypothermia has been estimated to kill perhaps twenty-five thousand Americans a year. Men and women over seventy-five seem to be five times more likely to succumb to it than those under seventy-five, according to one report. A recently completed ten-year study of victims of hypothermia found that most people who freeze to death are intoxicated or without proper shelter. So, despite the custom, avoid alcohol, particularly at bedtime. Hypothermia is also more likely to claim persons taking drugs, such as sleeping pills, some tranquilizers, even aspirin—all of which cause body temperature to drop.

How do you recognize hypothermia? Some warning signs include blueness or puffiness of the skin, slurred speech, poor coordination, confused behavior, dilated pupils, slowed breathing rate, and a weak or irregular pulse.

To stave off hypothermia, put on a sweater even if you don't feel cold if the room temperature falls below 65 degrees. Use thermal underwear or leg warmers if need be.

If you notice signs of hypothermia in an older person, act promptly to warm him or her up—in a warm bed with plenty of blankets, or an efficient electric blanket. If the person insists on staying up, add clothing—layers of it, because the air in between the layers acts as insulation. Warm gloves or slippers should be worn, too, as well as some kind of hat. And get the person to move about; muscle activity produces more body heat.

Another winter caution: If you've been outside on a cold windy day—a 20-degree reading with winds at forty-five miles an hour is the same as 40 degrees below zero on a still day—frostbite can occur. Body tissues literally freeze; crystals of ice form between cells.

To stave off frostbite, dress properly, avoid overexertion and excessive perspiration, don't touch cold metal with your bare hands, and don't smoke or drink alcohol.

If you do get frostbite, do *not* rub the affected area with snow; despite old advice about doing so, rubbing with snow only delays rewarming the area. In fact, do not touch the frozen spot at all. Instead, rewarm the area with warm (not hot) wet towels or take a warm (not hot) bath. And no matter how mild a case you may have, see a doctor as soon as possible.

What's right about a proper British tea party?

The timing. If you're going to drink any caffeinated drink—coffee, tea, cocoa, or a cola—the late afternoon is the best time for your body to handle it.

Chronobiologists—scientists who study the body's cycles—have observed how wakefulness and sleep are governed by certain hormones. Some stimulate daytime alertness; others promote evening and nighttime relaxation.

Coffee and tea in the morning are temporary lifts that actually upset the body's cycles, as does caffeine at night. In fact, as Dr. Charles Ehret of the Argonne National Laboratory near Chicago points out, your morning coffee or tea can make you feel sleepy during the day and restless at night. In addition to upsetting your biological clock, caffeine has the effect of raising blood-sugar levels, which gives the drinker a boost, but this lasts only about an hour and a half, because the body reacts to the higher sugar level by secreting insulin, which lowers blood sugar and can give you a tired and letdown feeling.

Because the "alert" hormones peak at about teatime—3:30 to 4:00 P.M., usually—that is when caffeine drinks will do the most to perk you up and have the least upsetting effect on your body's cycle.

It is also a myth that coffee sobers a person up. The Food and Drug Administration says caffeine is at best a weak antagonist of the depressant effects of alcohol. So giving strong black coffee to someone who has drunk too much may provide a false sense of confidence, because it won't improve the person's functioning, thinking, reflexes—or driving ability.

Americans consume an average of more than 200 milligrams of caffeine daily, and as a result many suffer a host of ailments from dizziness, headaches, and neck tension to sleeplessness, agitation, and irregular heartbeat. In other cases, reported in the journal *Postgraduate Medicine*, symptoms vary from diarrhea to cramps. Caffeine may also cause birth defects if pregnant women drink it in substantial amounts.

So gradually try to limit your intake. Don't go cold turkey—that can disrupt the cycle and cause caffeine-withdrawal headaches. Get yourself down eventually to a cup a day—and have it at teatime.

Should you smoke pot?

Not if you can help it. Virtually everyone should avoid it—for a variety of medical and legal reasons. Clearly, anyone who has a known heart or lung problem, such as atherosclerosis, or asthma with its complications in breathing, should avoid smoking pot. One joint is said to be capable of having the same effect upon the lungs as an entire pack of cigarettes. Pot can also boost a person's heart rate as much as 50 percent for a time.

Here are some other important warnings from medical experts:

☐ Don't use marijuana if you're pregnant. The major active ingredient in it—tetrahydrocannabinol, or THC—may influence the genetic machinery of living cells, including those of the fetus.

☐ If you're a teenager, keep in mind that marijuana may dull your mind and affect your hormonal system.

☐ Don't drive a car when under the influence. Your judgment may be impaired and accidents can result.

Marijuana may also trigger attacks in epileptics. And according to a report in the *Journal of the American Medical Association,* people with a tendency to schizophrenia or other mental problems may be driven out of control by marijuana.

Assessing or accepting claims about marijuana—good or bad—is clouded by emotions. Back in the 1930s, when the prohibition of alcohol was ending, some propaganda pictured marijuana—"dope," it was called then—as inciting murder, rape, robbery, incest, and a ticket to the loony bin. "Actual" case histories were cited that discouraged a generation or two of young people from using it. In the late 60s and early 70s, young people rediscovered marijuana, and found that most of the propaganda was exaggerated. But they went overboard in calling it safe and harmless. (And when the use of heroin became popular, too, many young people figured heroin dangers were also being exaggerated—which they weren't—and so got into deeper trouble.) At last count, one in nine high-school seniors was using pot daily and one fourth of our entire population had tried it.

Marijuana has its uses. It can be beneficial in relieving pain in the late stages of cancer; in fact, THC has been officially approved for this use. However, outside of supervised medical uses, marijuana is illegal—and the "grass" sold unlawfully, it should be pointed out, may contain harmful additives or impurities. It is, after all, not subject to any government standards or control.

Careful, objective medical-psychological studies are continuing to learn exactly what marijuana does. In the meantime, only people who need it medically should take it.

Is it healthy to feed a cold and starve a fever?

Not if you want to speed your recovery. Research has now found that any infection causes your body to burn more calories than normal—which means, the old adage notwithstanding, that for both you should eat *more* food and drink *more* liquids than normal. "Feed a cold, feed a fever" is now the slogan.

What should your cold menu include?

- [ ] Hot liquids. They tend to break up stuffy noses and relieve nasal congestion. Chicken soup seems to do it fastest. Moreover, if you're dizzy, salty liquids like chicken soup and bouillon can help.
- [ ] Water and other liquids—eight to twelve glasses a day, to avoid dehydration.
- [ ] Fruit juices. If you don't feel like eating, they'll provide the calories you need.

Here's what else you can do:

- [ ] Use a cool-air vaporizer or humidifier to help unclog nasal passages and cool a fevered person.
- [ ] Dress for comfort if you're suffering from a fever. Stay in bed and try to remain inactive. Wear light clothing and use a light sheet. Bundle up when you feel chills, but otherwise avoid excess clothing, which may actually drive body temperature higher.
- [ ] Use cool water rather than alcohol for sponging. Alcohol vapors can be dangerous, and the chilling effect of alcohol may be too sudden, causing the onset of severe chills.

Scientists have identified and isolated about two hundred viruses that can cause colds, but this is merely the tip of the iceberg. Although myths persist, there is still no folk remedy or medication available over the counter or through prescription that cures the common cold. In fact, a panel of nongovernment experts called together by the Food and Drug Administration to study fifty thousand cold, flu, cough, and allergy drugs found that the best some of these medicines could do was provide temporary relief from some cold symptoms. Moreover, the popular theory that vitamin C relieves colds has not been proved.

Many people rush to their doctors for a shot of penicillin or other antibiotic when they come down with a cold. Doctors sometimes administer these medicines just to appease the patient or to reduce the chances of secondary infection. But penicillin is not effective against colds, because colds are caused by viruses, not by the bacteria that penicillin kills.

Even the venerable aspirin, while still the most effective fever-reducing remedy, has come under criticism. A study conducted by the University of Illinois College of Medicine found that viruses grow more plentifully and for longer periods of time in the noses of cold sufferers who take aspirin. This may be because aspirin inhibits the production of interferon, one of the body's major virus-fighting substances. Aspirin, in fact, could be prolonging your cold rather than helping it.

The best cold and fever remedy is to get rest and more rest. Most colds are self-limiting and go away by themselves. If your cold persists, it's time to call your doctor.

Suffering from severe lower back pain? Ever hear of papaya?

There's a new treatment for slipped-disk sufferers, a drug, called chymopapain, that is derived from papaya. If you've tried bed rest and traction without success, and now you're contemplating surgery, think about trying chymopapain (marketed under the trade name Chymodiactin). It may be the answer for your aching back.

A slipped or herniated disk results from bulging of the inner portion of an intervertebral disk in the spine, which presses on the sciatic nerve, causing severe back, hip, and especially leg pain. Chymopapain, injected into the disk, dissolves the herniated material, thus relieving the pressure. (In surgery, the bulging material is cut away.)

Actually, chymopapain isn't new. It has been in use in Canada and elsewhere for twenty years, but it was not approved in the United States by the Food and Drug Administration until recently. Reasons for questioning its efficacy included the possibility of technical errors in carrying out the studies, and the use of an active placebo.

Canadian orthopedic surgeon John McCulloch, who has treated more than 4,500 people with the method, determined through careful study that chymopapain does not work for other than herniated disk conditions. It will not, for example, relieve back trouble caused by bone spurs, degenerative disk disease, or emotional stress. But for those with herniated disks, trials in the United States and elsewhere have shown a success rate varying from 59 percent to 80 percent, depending upon the criteria used. (Most failures are still susceptible to surgical intervention.) In follow-up studies of those treated early on, the beneficial effects still lasted after several years.

There is a very slight risk of allergic shock reaction with the use of chymopapain, which can be countered. The percentage of those suffering ill effects is as low as or lower than that associated with surgery. A surgical procedure requires an average hospital stay of two weeks, as opposed to a stay of one and a half to three days with chemonucleolysis, as the chymopapain-injection procedure is called. Outpatient treatment in a single day is currently being evaluated.

If you think chymopapain may help, check with an orthopedic or neurological surgeon to find out where to go for treatment.

When is imbibing healthy?

When your head is clear but your arteries may not be.

It's sensible to be concerned about the effects of drinking on your health. Alcohol is a leading contributor to illness and premature death. But if it's your heart that you're worried about, a little alcohol may actually be good for you.

According to recent studies at the National Heart Institute and elsewhere that involved sample groups of men matched for risk factors, those who regularly had one or two drinks a day had a lower incidence of coronary heart disease than the teetotalers. It didn't matter if the drinks were beer, wine, or hard liquor.

Coronary heart disease, which can lead to heart attacks, results when cholesterol deposits build up in the arteries that supply the heart muscle and diminish blood flow to the heart. Substances in the body called lipoproteins are involved in the process. There are good ones and bad ones. The good ones, high-density lipoproteins (HDL), work as scavengers, removing cholesterol deposits. They may also block the action of low-density lipoproteins (LDL), which are the bad ones, because they fill cells with fatty deposits. Alcohol *increases* HDL levels and *lowers* LDL levels.

Do these reports mean that we should all start drinking to save our hearts? Absolutely not. It simply means that very moderate drinkers may be at somewhat lower heart risk than total abstainers—though other factors, such as personality and lifestyle, may account for the difference.

What deadly toxin straightens crossed eyes?

The food poisoning known as botulism.

About sixty thousand people have surgery each year to correct crossed eyes. About half of them are considered candidates for a treatment, now in use in six centers in the United States and four abroad, that utilizes the neurotoxin botulin.

Botulism kills up to two thirds of its victims, usually through respiratory paralysis or secondary pneumonia. And it weakens eye muscles until recovery is complete.

Acting on that effect, Dr. Alan B. Scott, associate director of the Smith-Kettlewell Institute of Visual Sciences in San Francisco, found that by injecting a tiny amount of Oculinum toxin, a derivative of botulinum A, into the extraocular muscle of the strong or "pulling" eye in cross-eyed people, the muscle became temporarily paralyzed, causing it to stretch and relax, while the muscle of the other eye pulled up the slack, and tightened. These two effects, he discovered, can often straighten out the crossed eyes.

The treatment is not dangerous. Dr. Scott uses only one billionth of a gram of toxin. He first anesthetizes the strong eye with drops, then uses a special small needle that picks up electrical activity from the muscle to guide the toxin injection into the correct spot. About 40 percent of his patients—aged three to eighty—have needed only one injection of Oculinum. Another 40 percent have needed two injections, the rest still more. Usually painless, the entire procedure takes only five to ten minutes.

It's relatively easy to achieve the first five to ten degrees of strabismus (cross-eyed) change, Dr. Scott reports. Further change takes additional injections. Many patients do get double vision for a time, and need to wear an eye patch to relieve headaches or other effects.

"The treatment," Dr. Scott points out, "is not as permanent as surgical correction in many cases, but most patients feel the ease of retreatment compensates for this. About half of them have had prior unsuccessful eye surgery, up to five operations to straighten the eye."

What epidemic can you handle at home?

Head lice. And don't feel embarrassed if your child becomes a victim and host to this parasite. Epidemics can and do break out, because the louse travels easily and has staying powers. Children can contract head lice from youngsters at school, in summer camp, or at other communal places. And the head lice, formally known as *Pediculus humanis capitis*, pick on adults, too.

The lice are so tiny they're hard to see. They hold on to hairs with hooklike claws and opposing thumbs at the end of each of their six legs. You might see them crawling about on the scalp if you parted hairs with wood applicator sticks or used a hand lens. But the lice give themselves away through their eggs, called nits, which are silvery white and shiny, somewhat resembling dandruff. But dandruff flakes off, and nits are difficult to pull off. They surround hair shafts and are usually found near the scalp. Head lice seem to prefer the nape of the neck and behind the ears, but they can also infest eyelashes, beards, and mustaches.

The lice are bloodsucking parasites, and therein often is your first clue that you are dealing with a problem—the biting causes itching, and the child scratches his or her head in response. So be suspicious and check for head lice if the youngster starts scratching.

Treatment is simple and sure, if carried out properly. Remove all clothing. Wash the hair with a special lice-treating shampoo (A-200 or RC Shampoo, available at drugstores). Shampoo again eight to ten days later, to kill off any newly hatched lice. That should do the trick for the hair. Be sure to use a strong disinfectant on combs and brushes.

As for clothing that might be infested with nits, wash in hot water and soap, dry-clean what isn't washable, or seal the clothing up in an airtight plastic bag for ten days, long enough to kill the lice. Bedding, hair ribbons, hats, and scarves can be dealt with in this way. But the lice might have also invaded headrests and the backs of upholstered chairs, or auto seats, so clean them, too. This is one itch you don't want to have every seven years—or ever.

What's the point of visiting the dentist once you've lost 'em all?

To keep smiling and stay healthy. Unfortunately, too many elderly people figure there's no point to seeing a dentist once they've started to wear dentures; as many as 70 percent of them haven't been back to the dentist in five years. But they're wrong; they should see their dentist once a year.

Dentures need inspection. They could be irritating the gums, inducing sores and tumors in the mouth. Poorly fitting dentures can damage the jaw joint and speed the loss of supporting bone.

What denture wearers overlook is the fact that the shape of the mouth changes, albeit slowly. The supporting bone recedes about two millimeters every five to eight years. And that is bound to affect a patient's appearance, causing deep wrinkles around the mouth, or a thin-lipped look, or a jutting chin or pronounced lower jaw pouches. As a result, most dentures need to be replaced in time.

Between regular checkups, a denture wearer can help cut down on bone loss and keep the mouth healthy by consciously chewing straight up and down with equal weight on both sides of the jaw. Sideways chewing or favoring one side of the mouth can make dentures slip and lead to excessive wear.

The denture wearer also needs to brush the soft tissues beneath the denture to stimulate blood circulation and keep the gums healthy. Then, too, the denture should be removed for about eight hours every day. And when a denture breaks or comes loose, the wearer shouldn't try to fix it but rather should see a dentist.

There are dentists who specialize in elderly patients. To find one, write to the American Society for Geriatric Dentistry, 1121 W. Michigan Street, Indianapolis, IN 46202, enclosing a stamped, self-addressed envelope.

Who's often overlooked in a divorce?

Grandma and Grandpa. We all know how painful divorce can be for parents and children, but grandparents, too, are at a loss when they find themselves cut off abruptly from their grandchildren. The tragedy is that they could be a help to both their children and their children's children.

Grandparents often suffer when their children divorce. They can feel hurt or feel that they've somehow failed. And they can become resentful and distance themselves from their children and grandchildren—with painful results for all concerned.

Divorce can bring with it an almost infinite number of situations and regroupings, all of them sensitive. Parents with custody, for example, can in some states forbid the parents of a former spouse to see the grandchildren.

If grandparents are kept informed about a marriage in trouble, they are often sensitive to the feelings involved and can be helpful in offering the grandchildren a sense of continuity and an example of stability. More than half the states now have statutes that permit grandparents to petition the courts for visitation rights. And many lawyers now advise that a divorce agreement include a provision about the rights of all grandparents involved.

Some experts think that one way to alleviate the pain of a family breakdown is to add new members. They suggest that grandparents be brought into the household after a divorce—frequently, if not permanently—so that the children can benefit and develop more fully by exposure to a third generation.

What beat do babies rock to?

The sweetest music of all, and the first they ever hear—the beat of a loving heart.

Close your eyes and imagine a woman holding an infant, or visualize your favorite painting of a madonna and child. Chances are that the mother in your mind is cuddling her baby with her left arm. Research has shown that most women tend to this position. And they do it whether they're right- or left-handed. Anthropologists have observed this behavior among women in modern hospitals as well as in primitive tribal huts, and in mother-child depictions in the art of many cultures.

Some say mothers know instinctively that their heartbeats are calming and reassuring to their babies; others say that women have learned by trial and error that it's a practice that works. What about men? Do they have the same tendency? Apparently not. Ralph Bolton, an anthropologist at Pomona College in Claremont, California, who has studied the question, suggests that because in most societies it's the mother who has primary child-care responsibility, men just don't get the chance to learn the trick.

American society is fast changing into one in which both parents are more and more sharing the joys of bringing up baby. So, Dad, if you're holding a wailing infant, take it to heart. It would be a crying shame to miss the opportunity.

What's the hidden danger in a diaper change?

Powder. That seemingly innocent stuff you pat on your baby's tushy is responsible for thousands of accidents each year.

Most parents are alert to the poison dangers from household cleansers and drugs and keep them well out of the reach of curious toddlers. But few realize that even a baby under close parental supervision can still have a serious poisoning accident.

Here's a typical case. It's nearly dinnertime and you're in a hurry to get the diaper changed as quickly as possible; the baby is fussing, so you give her the bottle of talc to play with. The danger—your baby may swallow or inhale the powder. The symptoms are coughing, wheezing, choking, shortness of breath, even vomiting. And while the particles from the powder may not be poisonous in themselves, according to the National Poison Control Network, they are a foreign body that may trigger pneumonia and other lung problems if they are inhaled.

The network makes the following suggestions for protecting your infant at diapering time:

- ☐ Use petroleum jelly instead of talcum powder. It's nontoxic and does just as good a job of keeping the infant dry.
- ☐ Ointments used for an infant's rear end, and especially for diaper rash, contain zinc and should be treated as potentially dangerous because of zinc salts in them that a baby might ingest.
- ☐ Changing tables are built with mother's comfort and convenience in mind, not the infant's safety, so the lower the surface of the changing table, the better off the baby'll be, because the infant will have a shorter distance to fall. Plan ahead and make sure you have everything you need within easy reach so you won't be distracted from the baby.
- ☐ Give your baby a toy to keep him or her distracted while you change a diaper. But make sure the toy is safe. Check that it is too large to be swallowed and sturdy enough not to be dismantled and swallowed.
- ☐ Don't overlook the most obvious hazard—diaper pins. Don't leave one open and lying around on the changing table. If a closed pin is swallowed, chances are it will pass through the digestive system without a problem. However, if it is swallowed open, t could be dangerous. You should notify your pediatrician at once.

Do trust and gullibility go hand in hand?

No. Encouraging trust is an effective means of *preventing* gullibility. The child who trusts is able to discriminate between who is and isn't to be trusted.

The results of a fourteen-year study led by psychologist Dr.

Julian B. Rotter of the University of Connecticut strongly suggest that "high trusters" are no more likely to be led down the garden path than "low trusters." What's more, high trusters tend to be happier, better adjusted, and more popular than low trusters. The former are also perceived by others as more trustworthy themselves—and they are. The study showed that high trusters succumb much less frequently than low trusters to the temptation to lie, cheat, or steal when there is no risk of detection and punishment.

How do children develop trust and trustworthiness? Predictably, parents are the primary model. To teach trust, show that you can be trusted—and that it's a two-way street. If you tell your daughter you'll take her skating on Saturday if she completes her homework, take her—but only if she has fulfilled her part of the bargain. If you promise your son you'll pick him up at his friend's house at five, be there at five—and expect him to be ready to go.

Encourage a child's reasonable requests to take on more responsibility.

How can Chinese food be good for your health?

Maybe because of black tree fungus, a common ingredient of Chinese dishes like moo shu pork, hot and sour soup, and Szechwan hot bean curd. This squishy rubbery fungus, also known as tree ears, is served to add texture to dishes, but it may add years to one's life by preventing heart attacks. How? By keeping blood from clotting.

The theory is that of Dr. Dale E. Hammerschmidt, a blood specialist at the University of Minnesota Medical School in Minneapolis. An experiment of his was ruined when blood platelets taken from one man surprisingly failed to clump normally. Intrigued, the doctor tracked down the cause to the man's most recent meal, Szechwan hot bean curd. Testing indicated that the fungus in the bean curd was causing the blood to temporarily clot very slowly.

Dr. Hammerschmidt speculates that a chemical in tree ears, as yet not fully identified, is responsible; so far, it's known that the chemical is mostly adenosine. Chronic consumption of the fungus, he adds, "may contribute to the observed low incidence of atherosclerotic disease [in southern China] and thus explain the reputation of this fungus as a longevity tonic."

In China, tree ears are employed as a folk remedy for a wide array of ailments, including headaches, dysentery, and bleeding hemorrhoids. Other foods may also contain substances that have similar effects on the blood. Among them: ginger, mackerel, salmon, scallions, and garlic. These are being investigated by researchers studying heart disease.

All these findings are still theoretical, but until all the results are in, you can't go wrong with a dish from column A and another from column B.

How can eating help you drive from Dallas to Detroit?

Hearty meals in the midst of a long drive will help a driver maintain reaction time. Resting helps, but eating is important too.

Reactions slow the longer a driver keeps going, but researchers at the University of Uppsala, Sweden, report that reaction time slows less when drivers eat during a break. The length of the break doesn't matter.

During the Swedish test, drivers spent a total of eight hours on a freeway. They rested for either fifteen minutes or one hour after the first four hours of driving. Some of them ate a solid meal of meatballs, potatoes, bread and butter, and milk; others ate nothing. The results:

1. The reaction time of the drivers who ate was better than that of those who did not eat. Whether the drivers gulped their meals down in fifteen minutes or spent a leisurely hour eating, they outperformed the drivers who ate nothing.
2. The better performance occurred gradually over the long haul, however. Curiously, the drivers who ate did not experience an immediate pick-me-up.
3. The slower reaction time of the drivers who did not eat was the same whether they rested for fifteen minutes or for an hour.

Eating a big meal will not, of course, solve all the hazards of long-distance driving. An unrelated study also conducted at the

University of Uppsala concluded that nighttime driving breaks were less effective than daytime ones. Moreover, younger drivers recouped faster than older drivers.

So if you're going to be on the road for a long period of time, try to drive during daylight hours and eat a hearty meal. You'll feel better and be able to drive more safely.

Who misses the kids most when they move out?

More often than not, it's probably Dad.

Everyone assumes that Mom, especially if she's been home-bound, will suffer a severe emotional wrench when the nest empties out. After all, her main preoccupation for nearly twenty years has been the feeding, nurturing, and caring of the children. Now that they're gone, what would possibly keep her busy?

Well, surprise—sociologists and psychologists are finding that many women then feel a sense of relief and freedom—freedom to do all those things they've always wanted to do and never had the time for. They finally can think of enjoying time to themselves.

In one study of 160 women whose children were about to go off on their own, or already had done so, Lilian B. Rubin, a research sociologist at the Institute for the Study of Social Change, University of California at Berkeley, found that some of the women "were *momentarily* sad, lonely, or frightened of an uncertain future without kids, but they were not depressed. All except one responded to the actual or impending departure of their children with decided relief."

This particular analysis concerned white women aged thirty-five to fifty-four in the working, middle, and professional classes. All had given up careers after having worked for at least three years before becoming mothers and housewives. They had subordinated their personal dreams and wants, so "it is not surprising that when day-to-day care ends and the children leave, relief comes."

Dad, on the other hand, may feel an enormous sense of loss mixed with guilt. He thinks back over how often he didn't have time for the kids when they were young. And he can't bring their childhood back.

Fortunately, the times they seem to be a-changing. With more and more women choosing careers, fathers are showing a willingness to become increasingly involved with day-to-day child rearing. They are choosing participation now instead of regret later. Obviously, the best cure for the empty-nest syndrome is to start planning for it early.

Cellulite—fad or flab?

Medical and government authorities say that "cellulite"—those dimply bulges that collect on the thighs and buttocks of thousands upon thousands of despairing women—is just plain flab.

If you've heard that cellulite is something unique, a buildup of toxins and wastes that you can get rid of only with special creams, massages, or other treatments, forget it. "There is no medical condition known or described as cellulite in this country," says the *Journal of the American Medical Association.* When doctors look at "cellulite" under a microscope, what they see is ordinary fat.

Certain body cells have the ability to hold enormous amounts of fat. Fat has to be stored someplace, and people vary in their characteristic storage depots. These variations tend to run in families. In addition, men generally park their excess poundage around their middle, while women often carry it well below the belt. The unhappy result is frequently what's become known as cellulite: fat deposits on the thighs and fanny that get their "orange peel" appearance from overstuffed fat cells that bulge up just beneath the skin surface.

What can you do about the hard-to-budge pudge? The U.S. Food and Drug Administration warns that the first thing you should do is ignore any claims about special treatments that get rid of those lumps. Hang on to the money you were planning to spend on special sponges, washcloths, mitts, creams, vitamin-mineral supplements, books, bath liquids, massagers, rubberized pants, brushes, rollers, and toning lotions. Stay away also from salon treatments, which are equally worthless—and costly.

Does that mean you can't get rid of cellulite? Not at all. Obesity experts advise using exactly the same tactics as you would on any other body bulges: exercise and a carefully balanced weight-loss diet.

When are sunglasses the answer?

Summer *and* winter.

The glare of reflected sunlight on snow and ice, or on a long stretch of highway, can be just as dangerous as summer sun on sand and sea.

Continuous unprotected exposure to the ultraviolet rays of bright sunlight can severely damage the cornea, the transparent outer covering of the eyeball. That's one major reason for the tens of thousands of serious eye injuries traced each year to recreational activities alone—and most of them could have been prevented. The longer, more frequent the exposure, the greater the risk.

A less critical but very common result of going without sunglasses is burns on the sensitive skin around the eyes. You know how it is. You're at the beach, you lie back and close your eyes, and off come the shades. After all, who wants big white rings like an owl? Put them back on or you may wind up looking a good deal worse.

And if the weather's bad but you're still determined to tan with a sunlamp, even sunglasses are not good enough. You'll need special goggles.

When buying sunglasses, select a style that is fairly large and close-fitting. The lenses should be gray, green, or brown for the best protection and least distortion. Put them on and look in the mirror. If you can still see your eyes, they're not dark enough. Check if there is a label on the glasses that tells the percentage of light transmission. For use in heavy sun, the less the better: no more than 15 percent. For average sun, 30 to 35 percent.

Skiers and sailors should consider wearing polarized or mirrored lenses, which greatly reduce snow and water glare. Phototropic lenses, which adjust to varying light, are versatile; they're also more expensive.

If you normally wear corrective lenses, prescription sunglasses are better than the kind you clip over your regular glasses.

To check the quality of sunglass lenses, hold them about ten inches from your eyes and look through them at a square edge. The image shouldn't wiggle when you move them from side to side.

Don't make the mistake of going to the other extreme and

wearing sunglasses when you don't need them. Indoors, and when the sun goes down, the sunglasses should come off. Otherwise you will not have enough light to see properly. And young children shouldn't wear sunglasses—which can break during play and cause injuries—unless they are extremely sensitive to light and their doctor advises it.

If you've been exposed, unprotected, to strong sunlight and suffer sharp pain or a grainy feeling in the eyes later, even a day later, it is important to get medical attention immediately. Be sure to consult an ophthalmologist, who specializes in eye disorders. The neighborhood optician or optometrist is not qualified to deal with such problems. Seeing a doctor quickly reduces the chance of permanent injury. If you're wise, you won't take the chance at all.

Should you push your preschooler to make friends?

Never. Friendships among young children should occur naturally. Putting a lot of pressure on children to make friends can result in obsessive concern about popularity that will last into later life. Such children don't develop their own individuality, and they conform too much to the standards of their playmates.

Different children have different social needs and styles, including a real need on the part of many children for privacy and solitude. And the quality of social relationships is more important than quantity.

While you should avoid pushing, you should be willing to encourage your child's friendships; they serve many important functions, just as they do in adults. Friendships help a young child to communicate more successfully, and also aid in learning social skills, especially those dealing with resolving conflicts. Having friends the same age will also help children learn to compare themselves with each other, not for competitive reasons, but as a way of beginning to develop a sense of their own identity. Moreover, friendships foster the sense of belonging to a group, a critical need for all human beings.

Children begin to have a capacity for friendship shortly after the age of two, but they are usually awkward about it at first. However, parents can smooth the way. Family Focus, a Chicago-area program that provides drop-in support centers for parents of children who are three or under, points out that:

☐ When children are just beginning to play with others, it's easier for them to have one playmate at a time for a while. Many children also enjoy small play groups that can add interest and fun. Play groups work best when adults plan ahead and provide an absorbing activity such as using crayons or clay.

☐ Playing with other children also requires that each child have time to observe and to find his or her own way of playing. Some youngsters assume the role of leader, others of follower, while still other children enjoy observing from the sidelines or, in some cases, initiate a noisy activity. A child who is passive at one time can emerge as assertive another.

☐ Two-year-olds cannot yet organize their play together. They still require an adult who is alert to when things get rambunctious—noise and chaos are scary to young children. The adult should be on hand to settle disputes and to help children learn to share and to be aware of each other's feelings.

☐ Between two and three years of age, the child makes leaps forward in social ability, though still playing alone a great deal. The youngster also wants to be with children of the same age and older, often liking to imitate older children and learning by doing so.

Keep in mind that while learning the art of friendship is a crucial part of growing up, every child is unique and will have individual ways of playing with friends.

How low can low back pain get?

Would you believe as low as your feet? The causes of low back pain—an ailment that afflicts 60 percent of the working population at one time or another—are many and sometimes mysterious. But a portion of the half million cases treated annually may be due not to problems in the lower back itself but rather to problems with the feet.

Flat feet, which sometimes runs in families, can result in abnormal posture. That, in turn, leads to ill-defined low back pain and fatigue, and also sciatica. (The sciatic nerve, the largest and longest in the body, originates in the lower part of the spine and descends along the back of the leg. Sciatica usually manifests itself as a pain, sometimes severe, down the back of the thigh.)

The opposite of flat feet, very high arches, can also cause chronic back pain and a sciatica-like pain. In addition, slight differences between the two feet can result in back pain, by causing one leg to be a little longer than the other.

Certain shoes can cause back problems, too. Very small differences in heel heights between a right shoe and a left shoe can contribute to back pain, and to its relief. Paying attention to how your back feels when you wear a particular pair of shoes can be the first step toward helping you relieve it. Discard shoes that make your back hurt. If your back hurts no matter what shoes you wear, modifying your shoes with lifts or inserts can sometimes change your posture or the tilt of your pelvis enough to bring blessed relief. As researchers at Iowa State University found, the muscles and skeletal systems of some people with low back pain don't do a good job of absorbing the bone vibrations set off every time their heels hit the ground. The simple solution: flexible arch supports, the kind you find at the drugstore. Of eighty-one patients who tried them, 60 percent were pain-free within a month, and 90 percent within a year. But before you do-it-yourself, check with your doctor.

Can vitamin C *cause* scurvy?

Yes, if you suddenly stop taking it after you've been ingesting large doses for a while. The condition is known as "rebound scurvy."

It's been known for centuries that small amounts of vitamin C prevent scurvy, a painful disease that leads to bleeding gums and loose teeth. British sailors took vitamin C–containing limes to eat on long voyages to prevent the disease—and got the nickname "limeys."

Recently, however, doctors have begun to diagnose scurvy in people who've been taking large amounts of vitamin C in the hope of preventing colds and then quit suddenly, perhaps because their supply ran out. They've found rebound scurvy not only in adults who abruptly stopped taking vitamin C but also in infants born to women who took megadoses of the vitamin during pregnancy.

Most people who believe vitamin C will lessen their chances of catching cold take at least 1,000 milligrams a day, and often more. When a person does so, the body must speed up its method of eliminating the excess, and the accelerated rate, according to Robert L. Pollack, a nutrition expert at Temple University in Philadelphia, "persists even after the patient stops taking the vitamin. As a result, essential vitamin C may be washed out of the system and cause damage to the oral tissues."

He recommends that people take no more than 100 to 200 mg of vitamin C daily. And if you're already taking megadoses, taper off instead of quitting cold turkey.

Is it wise to pull that wisdom tooth?

It's the wisest thing you can do with a problem tooth, dental surgeons say.

Wisdom teeth, it turns out, are very nearly vestigial. The bigger jaws of our early ancestors could handle those extra molars, but today our jaws are too small. The result: There often isn't room enough for wisdom teeth to grow in straight, or to take their place without crowding their neighbors.

The 3,500-member American Association of Oral and Maxillofacial Surgeons says the chances that impacted wisdom teeth will straighten themselves out and not cause trouble are slight.

Wisdom teeth got their name because they normally come through the gums during adolescence, when we are supposedly wising up about the world. Our jaws are fully developed then.

In nine out of ten people, at least one wisdom tooth becomes trapped or impacted in the gum, able only to breach the surface slightly. A partly exposed wisdom tooth is subject to dental decay. Gum tissues are vulnerable to infection and inflammation; damaging cysts may form underneath.

The conventional wisdom used to be to leave wisdom teeth alone until they hurt. Not anymore. It's been found that people who wait till their forties to have wisdom teeth removed have problems at least four times as serious as those who had the extractions in their twenties.

The National Institutes of Health gathered together three hundred orthodontists, oral surgeons, and dentists for a conference, and they came to a consensus on two points:

☐ Crooked or impacted wisdom teeth are an abnormal condition that in itself may justify removal.

☐ Complications during or after surgery may be reduced if impacted wisdom teeth are removed in the mid-teens, when the roots are not yet fully formed and the bone around them is less dense than it will be at maturity.

Many dental surgeons advise parents to have their children's teeth X-rayed between the ages of eight and twelve to see which, if any, of the wisdom teeth are going to come in straight—and to be prepared to have the others removed between the ages of fifteen and twenty-one. Doing it can save pain and money later on.

━━━━━━━━━━━━━━

What's the peril in a pot of herb tea?

It can be a health bomb. Touted as health foods, many herbs are actually drugs affecting both body and mind.

Some popular herb teas can kick up blood pressure and heart rate, bring on dizziness, cramps, and diarrhea, cause hallucinations and other mental or emotional effects, and endanger unborn babies.

Such effects should not be surprising, considering that mankind's very first medicines were all from herbs and other plants. Quinine, used to combat malaria, comes from the bark of the cinchona shrub; digitalis, the heart stimulant, is a derivative of foxglove; colchicine, to combat gout, comes from meadow saffron. Today, nearly half of all prescription drugs contain active ingredients extracted from or first detected in plants.

Herbal teas, says Dr. Ara Der Marderosian, are "crude complexes containing many impurities and active components with a variety of possible undesirable effects. Some are actually too dangerous to be used at all." Dr. Der Marderosian is professor of pharmacognosy—the science of drugs of natural origin—at the Philadelphia College of Pharmacy and Science.

Another medical expert warns that some herbal teas used in excess may cause harm. They are "not substances to be used frivolously."

Some of the dangerous herbs in teas include chamomile, mistletoe, senna, nutmeg, sassafras, and jimson weed. One woman drinking nutmeg tea became incoherent and giddy. Hallucinations overcame a young man drinking tea made from jimson weed. Teas from mint and chamomile can stimulate contractions of the uterus early in pregnancy, threatening miscarriages. Ginseng tea may stimulate the adrenal glands and thyroid gland, making your heart race. Some ingredients in herbal teas may conflict with or counteract the activity of prescription drugs.

Herbal teas may contain just one active ingredient or be a blend of as many as twenty different chemical agents from leaves, seeds, or flowers. Devotees sometimes urge friends to switch to herbs to avoid the caffeine in coffee or regular tea, or claim extraordinary health benefits from herbal teas. But drink with caution. The safest are red zinger, lemon balm, anise, rose hip, raspberry, and lemon grass. If in doubt, ask your doctor.

Is lead a booby trap for children?

It has been—but now there's a simple, inexpensive blood test to spot a harmful level.

For children, lead is one of the worst poisons. Even low levels in the body can damage nerves and the brain, the kidneys, and the blood-forming system.

It's so serious that one study estimates that 4 percent of American children between the ages of six months and five years—about 675,000 in all—have higher levels of lead in their blood than the amount considered a safe cutoff point. The survey, made by a team from the National Center for Health Statistics, also came up with the grim finding that black children and poor children were far more likely to have lead poisoning that could affect intellectual and behavioral development. One in five black children under age five in inner cities has threatening amounts of lead. High levels were ten times more prevalent among poor children than those in the upper middle class.

The National Academy of Sciences estimates that about 600,000 tons of lead are added to our polluted environment each year through various uses of the metal. Countless additional tons are dispersed through the mining, smelting, manufacturing, and recycling of lead and lead-containing products.

Lead paint, a major threat for little children who may chew paint from windowsills and walls, is still present in many homes. More than half of all existing homes were built before 1960, and may contain lead paint. Children can also become poisoned from soil or dust saturated by lead from gasoline or factory smokestacks. An inner-city child can ingest 300 to 400 micrograms of lead just by licking his or her finger after playing outdoors; that's three to four times the daily amount considered safe.

Foods can contribute to unwanted lead, too. The Food and Drug Administration has issued an advisory warning that the amount in foods packaged in lead-soldered cans may increase if the food is not removed after the can has been opened. It reported studies finding that the longer orange juice is kept in a can the more lead it absorbs.

So repaint your home—starting with the nursery—with lead-free paint if you've got a toddler in the house. And if your child is between six months and five years old and you're at all concerned that he or she may have picked up too much lead from the environment, ask the doctor about the erythrocyte protoporphyrin screening test. It will not only identify lead exposure but also indicate whether your youngster has an iron deficiency.

What's the difference between reading a book and watching TV?

Reading a book uses less energy. Not *personal* energy; as we all know, sitting in front of the tube doesn't use much of that. Rather, the total energy cost of manufacturing a TV set is much greater than the energy cost of publishing a book. Thus, TV watching is more energy-intensive, or energy-consuming. And, surprisingly, it turns out that people are more likely to be content when they are engaging in an activity that has consumed little energy than they are when pursuing one that has consumed a lot.

Researchers at the University of Chicago decided to test the assumption, common in developed societies, that engaging in energy-intensive activities produces more happiness. They studied 107 people, but found no positive relationship between energy use and happiness. In fact, the women in their study were less happy when involved in high-energy-consuming activities. Many people are happier, it turns out, when they are daydreaming, participating in sports, or engaging in sexual activity—all low on the energy-consumption scale.

Why? The scientists think the key to happiness in an activity may be involvement. Energy-consuming activities are often passive activities, requiring very little input from the people engaged in them. (One exception: going out to a restaurant or disco. These are high-energy activities, but they also rate high on the happiness scale, perhaps because they call for active participation.)

The researchers conclude that, in our attempts to make our lives easier through intensive use of energy, from blenders to speedboats, we actually may have taken much of the joy out of life because we also, inadvertently, have reduced our active involvement. Want to be happy? Scuttle the speedboat and dive into a good book.

Do pesticides still affect our food?

To some extent, yes, but tainting is now rare. Still, if you're concerned, there are ways to reduce the incidence to a minimum.

Every day Americans eat tons of food carrying traces of pesticides, many of which have caused serious health hazards in animal testing. But those cases of pesticide poisoning that are reported mainly involve people exposed to large doses—chemical and farm workers, and small children who have access to improperly stored household pesticides.

Pesticides are used because they reduce crop losses due to pests. The cosmetic result is appealing, unscarred produce. But before a pesticide can be sold or used, a safe level of residue on food must be established. By the time the produce reaches market, most of the pesticide has either been washed off or has evaporated. Residues may remain, however, both on the surface of the food and inside it. Moreover, the label "organically grown" is no guarantee that the produce is free of pesticides—although it usually means they cost a lot more.

Growing your own food won't eliminate health problems if you live in a city or manufacturing area, because the air in your neighborhood and the water you use might be contaminated by heavy metals such as lead that have infiltrated natural resources.

And systemic pesticides—those that plants absorb through their roots or leaves into their tissues—can pose a hazard for inexperienced gardeners, who sometimes misuse them by overspraying or by spraying food plants with pesticides that are intended for use only on ornamentals such as flowers, shrubs, and trees.

Here's what you can do to reduce exposure to pesticide residues:

☐ Wash all fruits and vegetables carefully, preferably with biodegradable detergent. If you don't want to use soap, try soaking the produce for five minutes in a mixture of ¼ cup vinegar and 1 gallon of water. Then rinse thoroughly in cold water.

☐ Peel all fruits and vegetables. This is especially important for fruits such as apples and pears.

☐ Cook your vegetables in addition to peeling them. This and peeling usually get rid of 90 percent of pesticide residues.

☐ Eat lean red meat, trimming off any fat. Cook the meat well. (Pesticides lodge in fatty tissue.)

Though not all pesticide residues can be eliminated or are necessarily harmful in minute amounts, it's obviously healthy to remove as many as you can.

Which cancer in men is curable?

The one men probably fear most, testicular cancer.

The fear is not justified, doctors say. When caught early, testicular cancer is curable in at least eight of every ten cases. The treatment: surgery to remove the affected testicle combined with radiation or drugs to knock out residual malignant cells. A man's potency should remain undiminished, and if only one testicle has been removed so should his fertility.

According to researchers, men stand a greater risk of developing the disease if they have a testicle that has not descended into the scrotum. This condition, called cryptorchidism, occurs in 1 out of every 400 to 500 boys, and doctors recommend that a simple operation be performed at age two or three to correct the condition. If the surgery is delayed beyond age six, however, the chances of developing testicular cancer rise by 10 to 40 percent.

As with breast cancer, the best course is early detection. Doctors advise that all men, starting at age fifteen, examine their testicles monthly. The self-exam is simple to do. Take a hot shower to relax the muscles in the scrotum. Then, holding the testicle between the index finger and thumb, gently roll it, feeling for smoothness and firmness. Any lump, enlargement, or increased hardness in the testicle (as opposed to the various ducts and cords that lead to and from the scrotum) should be checked out with a doctor.

Can sterilization in a woman be reversed?

Yes, in many cases—and so can vasectomy in a man.

For years sterilization was regarded as an irreversible operation. That had been considered one of its advantages. By permanently blocking the fallopian tubes—the ducts in which sperm and egg unite—a woman was spared the muss and fuss and continual worry that plague other birth-control measures like the diaphragm, the pill, and condoms. Indeed, sterilization is the most prevalent form of birth control among both men and women throughout the world; 100 million couples had resorted to it as of 1980.

Today, though, more and more women want to have the operation reversed. The main reason for the trend: the growing incidence of divorce and remarriage. Many embarking on their second or third marriage want to have children with their new spouse. Luckily, doctors can offer considerable hope about reversing the operation.

The key is microsurgery. With the aid of high-power microscopes that magnify the fallopian tubes, surgeons are able to see the tissue in detail and do delicate stitching using sutures finer than a human hair to reconstruct the passages. A study at the Johns Hopkins School of Medicine showed that of twenty-six women who had microsurgery to reverse sterilization operations done an average of seven years before, seventeen, or 63 percent, were able to conceive and carry to term.

The reversal of a vasectomy is accomplished in similar fashion. The vas deferens—the tube carrying sperm—is reopened by microsurgery. The success rate ranges from 15 to 70 percent.

The success of the reversal operations is largely dependent on how much damage was done to the ducts in the original sterilization. Doctors stress that microsurgical reversal is a lengthy and expensive operation. In a woman, it also increases the risk of having an ectopic or tubal pregnancy.

If you're thinking of being sterilized, above all don't consider it a temporary birth-control measure. A reversal is possible but not at all guaranteed.

When's a good time to leave the TV set on?

When you know what your children are watching—or, better yet, when you're watching with them, which can be a positive learning experience for the youngsters.

The catalogue of criticisms of TV is a thick one. There's violence—as many as five violent acts an hour on prime-time television, eighteen violent acts an hour on children's weekend programming, according to the National Institute of Mental Health. The U.S. Surgeon General's Office, among others, believes such violence results in violent behavior by children and adults.

Another common activity that is often, and unrealistically, presented on TV is drinking; no matter what the hour or the situation, there will most likely be some form of alcohol present. Then, too, few television heroes are minority persons, and most authority figures are white men. And mentally ill characters are often depicted as violent or as the victims of violence.

The average preschool child watches 33 hours of television a week; schoolchildren under twelve watch an estimated 29 hours. A study by the State University of New York found that young people now finishing high school will have spent 16,500 hours in school and 20,500 hours watching TV.

What can you do? First of all, take charge of the set. Realistically, you have to acknowledge that TV is an important part of people's lives. But you can demystify it by explaining to your children and discussing with them the difference between animated and live action. You can point out special TV effects and teach them that the purpose of commercials is to enhance products, not to show life as it really is.

When you watch programs with your child, you can compare them with real life. For example, are the local police like TV police? Are the black families (and women, teachers, parents, and children) who are depicted like those they know? Explain how TV violence is often distorted and how they can't imitate it without suffering consequences that TV may not show.

Also, you can teach your children to be selective TV watchers by being one yourself. Use a TV schedule to choose programs instead of just turning on the set and letting it run. If your children are interested in a particular program, perhaps you can find books on the same subject.

Don't use television as an unmonitored baby-sitter. A child's mind is usually not at work when watching TV; he or she is merely a passive receiver.

Even educational programs are more effective when parents are watching too. And studies show that problems caused by watching television are rare in families that talk about what they're watching. So when you turn on the TV, make it a time for togetherness and talk, and you can also make it a time for learning.

The federal government publishes a free leaflet, "A Family Guide to Television," which you can get by writing Dept. 515H, Children and Television, Consumer Information Center, Pueblo, CO 81009.

When is home a hospital?

When someone needs care but doesn't have to be in a hospital or nursing home. For hundreds of thousands of people, that can often mean a more comfortable if not quicker recovery without sacrificing the quality of care. A less expensive one, too—and most health-insurance plans cover home-care services.

The American Public Health Association estimates that as many as one out of four patients now in hospitals or nursing homes could live at home with various kinds of aids. A study of its benefits in Connecticut found that home care led to an overall nine-day reduction in hospital stays, with an estimated savings of $4 million.

For those who do not need round-the-clock, seven-day-a-week supervision, home care has many benefits. Most important: familiar surroundings and the love of relatives and friends—vital ingredients for a healthy recovery.

Many people are not aware of the availability of home-care services—"one of the best-kept secrets around," says one health worker. But it needn't be. There are visiting nurses, Meals On Wheels programs, home-health aides, social workers, hospital outpatient services, ambulance services, and other programs—for therapy, counseling, tests, even shopping, cooking, and housework. And more than five thousand government, charitable, and commercial home-health-care agencies provide them.

To find out more, check with your doctor, the social-service director of a hospital, or your local Visiting Nurse Association, or look in the Yellow Pages under "Home Health Agencies." You can also write to the National Council for Homemaker–Health Aide Services, 67 Irving Place, New York, NY 10003, which maintains a nationwide list of home-care services; the National League for Nursing, 10 Columbus Circle, New York, NY 10019; or the Home Health Services and Staffing Association, Suite 205, 1101 15th Street NW, Washington, DC 20005, which lists proprietary services.

Does baby have to have your allergies?

Sneezing and wheezing have plagued your life, and perhaps your spouse is allergic, too. Is your youngster going to have to suffer the same miseries? Not necessarily. A child with allergic parents *is* more likely to develop allergies than a child whose family has been spared them. But even with a genetic predisposition, there's a good chance of escaping allergies. The odds are in your child's favor. Only sixteen out of a hundred children with a family history of allergy actually go on to become allergic themselves.

Furthermore, many doctors believe there are steps a parent can take to reduce the chances that a child will be saddled with allergies:

- ☐ If you're pregnant and also allergic, avoid foods that can trigger allergy attacks. Some doctors believe that during pregnancy allergies can get started in the developing fetus.
- ☐ If you're pregnant or nursing, avoid large amounts of eggs, milk, wheat, beef, chocolate, and nuts.
- ☐ Be careful also of the baby's diet. Breast-feeding is best, for at least six months, longer if possible. Cow's milk and milk products are powerful and common allergy triggers. Even soy substitutes don't always work, so check with your pediatrician if a problem develops.
- ☐ Delay the introduction of solid foods until six months. For the first year of life, don't feed your baby eggs, fish, chocolate, strawberries, or citrus juices.
- ☐ Fabrics can provoke allergies, so avoid woolen clothing and blankets. Some synthetics are also suspect. Use cotton when you can.
- ☐ Because pollen and other allergens can be spread by apparel, keep indoor and outdoor clothes in separate closets, and keep shoes separate, too, or wipe them clean before bringing indoors.
- ☐ Don't adopt a pet when pregnant. If you already have one, make Felix or Fido sleep outdoors if possible. Get rid of dust and mold in your home by damp-mopping often.
- ☐ Try to keep your baby from getting colds and other virus infections. They make asthma worse. Researchers at the University of California at San Francisco have discovered that minor virus infections during early infancy appear to trigger the first allergy attack in the children of allergic parents. Anyone with a cold or flu should stay away from the baby.
- ☐ If you smoke, stop. Children who live in households with smokers have more frequent and severe asthma attacks, and more respiratory symptoms, than children of smoke-free households. Besides, quitting will be good for *you*, too.

When is feeling sick good for you?

When you're pregnant, strangely enough. Nausea and vomiting are signs that the body is making necessary adjustments and that the fetus is growing. A curious corollary: Women who suffer morning sickness rarely miscarry.

The distress experienced by just about half of all expectant women in the first three months results from profound physical and chemical changes that stimulate the brain's nausea and vomiting center. Among the stimuli are the stretching of the uterine wall and the increased production of certain hormones. For example, the levels of progesterone and human chorionic gonadotropin (HCG) go up. These hormones relax muscle tissue and may slow the contractions of the stomach, delaying its emptying, leaving it uncomfortably distended, and creating an irritating reservoir of stomach acid.

For most women, the discomfort can be eased through simple means:

☐ Get plenty of rest. Sleep an extra two to four hours each night during early pregnancy.

☐ Take walks in the fresh air and do some light exercising.

☐ Eat small amounts in frequent feedings rather than three large meals. Try drinking a hot cup of tea and eating dry toast before getting out of bed in the morning, or as soon as you're up. Carry dry crackers around with you to nibble on when you feel nauseous.

☐ Avoid rich, greasy foods. Keep to simple baked or broiled meats, chicken, and fish.

☐ Check with your doctor about taking supplemental vitamin B_6.

If the nausea and vomiting persist to the point at which you are incapacitated, you may want to consider taking medication. But doctors caution that, in order to protect the fetus, pregnant women should take no drugs unless absolutely essential.

One drug once given almost routinely to expectant women to control nausea and vomiting—Bendectin—is no longer being manufactured. Over the past quarter century, more than 30 million women took it. Some researchers, as well as parents who have filed over two hundred lawsuits, believe that Bendectin could have caused birth defects. Yale University researchers recently reported that its use was linked to pyloric stenosis, a stomach defect in newborns. Although earlier an advisory committee of the Food and Drug Administration, after reviewing numerous previous studies, found no association between Bendectin and an increased risk of birth defects, it nevertheless added: "However, the committee felt that 'residual uncertainty' existed in spite of the largely negative human experience since it is not possible to prove unequivocally that a drug could never cause birth defects. The committee recommended continued monitoring."

The best advice is, if you can tough it out, avoid all drugs. And remember, morning sickness lasts only about three months.

How do you tell if you're too fat?

With a scale *and* a tape measure.

One of the most firmly documented medical facts is the relationship between weight and health. Studies such as the Framingham Heart Study and others by the American Cancer Society and insurance companies have monitored hundreds of thousands of men and women over many years. They all agree that the fatter you are, the more likely you are to get sick and die young. Even a few extra pounds can significantly increase the statistical risk. Slightly underweight, generally speaking, is healthier than slightly overweight. (The exceptions involve those who are smokers or who are underweight because of illness. The former are almost always the highest-risk group of all.)

Moreover, those who are fat early in life are likely to remain so as adults, which has led researchers to caution parents against overfeeding infants and children.

But what constitutes overweight? Clearly, cultural norms and personal taste (he likes Mae West and she likes Twiggy) influence our perception. In a survey at New York University, 20 percent of the men rated themselves—erroneously—as slightly underweight, while 69 percent of the women thought themselves overweight when only 39 percent were.

Optimal weight, say the experts, must be measured in pounds, inches, and the percentage of muscle and fat at any given height.

Generally speaking, an adult's weight should remain at what it was at age twenty-five, provided that at that age the person was in good shape. However, a sedentary life may bring on too much flab no matter what the scale says. A study matching men of equivalent weights and heights, half of them twenty-two years old and the other half forty-four, showed the older men to have twice as much body fat.

Take a tape measure. Does your waist measure six inches less than your chest? Ideally, it should be at least that for a man, about that for a woman (measured just below the bustline). Is your waistline *larger* than your chest? According to the Metropolitan Life Insurance Company, you can deduct two years from your life expectancy for every inch your waistline exceeds your chest.

The answer to creeping fat remains what it's always been: less calories and more exercises. A lifetime regimen of foods high in nutrients and low in calories—vegetables, fruit, complex carbohydrates, and lean protein—is the only miracle diet that works. Jogging, swimming, tennis, walking, and climbing stairs are all good ways to keep weight down and spirits high. For problem areas like a flabby stomach, you may need specific exercises such as sit-ups. Doctors, gyms, and health publications offer exercise plans. Ask about them.

One note of cheer comes from nutrition research conducted at the University of Michigan, which has shown that the obese become lean more often than the lean become obese. It's a good thought, but don't get carried away by it the next time there's chocolate mousse on the menu.

What's a gabber got to worry about?

His—or her—voice. A child who loudly and constantly mimics all the sound effects of, say, an airplane may be damaging the vocal cords.

Excessive talking, as well as yelling and screaming, is the most common causes of voice damage. Moreover, nervousness and tension can compound vocal abuse.

According to Dr. Morton Cooper of Los Angeles, a voice and speech therapist, each person has a natural or optimal pitch level within his or her voice that provides the most amount of sound for the least amount of effort. This optimal pitch level should be your habitual pitch level. If it isn't, you may be misusing your voice.

One way to check your pitch level is to say "um-hum" naturally. Then say "um-hum one," "um-hum two." Is the pitch of the "um-hums" the same as the numbers?

Another way, recommended by Dr. Cooper, is to place one hand on your chest and the other on your stomach. Breathe in with your stomach moving out while making a humming sound with your lips closed. Press in on your stomach in a quick staccato fashion. The sound—your habitual pitch—should escape from your nose, but you should feel a buzz around the mouth and nose.

The physical production of sound is the most rapid and complex of all muscular activities of our bodies. Hoarseness or laryngitis; a squeaky, foggy, breathy, or nasal voice; a voice that is too high or too low, too loud or too soft, or habitually breaks—all are indications of vocal-cord abuse and could lead to more serious medical problems.

Consistent vocal stress can lead to the development of a teardrop-shaped growth on the vocal cords called a polyp. Alternatively, scar tissue (or nodules) can form on the vocal cords. Infrequently, contact ulcerations or granuloma can develop. Generally all these are benign conditions that can be treated conservatively. Vocal rest is probably the simplest and most effective way to minimize vocal stress, but here are some other pointers on avoiding laryngitis or loss of voice:

- ☐ Always talk in a moderate tone and volume, even in noisy situations.
- ☐ Don't make a habit of screaming or yelling.
- ☐ If you smoke, stop. Cigarettes are a major cause of cancer of the larynx, of which the chief sign is hoarseness.
- ☐ Try to avoid being directly under or in front of an air-conditioning unit for long periods of time. (Home heating units can also dry out the air and cause vocal strain.)
- ☐ If stress is hurting your vocal cords, a simple relaxing exercise is to yawn and then sigh.

If vocal problems continue, however, voice therapy may be needed. In such cases, consult your doctor.

Does getting old have its advantages?

Yes, and one of the nicest is that it can save you money. If you're sixty-two or older and you want a sightseeing vacation, you can save yourself a tidy sum if you pack your camper, load up your knapsack, and visit our federal lands.

The U.S. government will issue you a Golden Age Passport that, for free, lets you and your traveling companion and your vehicle enter any federal park, recreation area, or monument that ordinarily charges an entrance fee. The passport also entitles you to a 50 percent discount on parking, boat launching, and camping. The only costs it doesn't cover are those charged by private concessionaires operating on the grounds.

How can you get a Golden Age Passport? Easily, as long as you get it in person; you can't write away for one. Bring proof of age—either a driver's license, a birth certificate, or a Medicaid card—to any of the following places: National Park Service and Forest Service Headquarters or regional offices; Forest Service Supervisor's offices; most Forest Service ranger station offices; all National Park System areas charging admissions; Bureau of Land Management state and district offices; Tennessee Valley Authority–Land between the Lakes, and all recreation areas that charge fees; all Fish and Wildlife Service regional offices and National Wildlife Refuges where Land and Water Conservation Fund use fees are in effect; and Bureau of Reclamation–Hoover Dam.

Because almost all the federally operated recreation areas keep a supply of passports on hand, you don't have to go to the trouble of getting one ahead of time. And it's good for life.

If you're not sixty-two but are blind or permanently disabled, you may qualify for a Golden Access Passport, a free lifetime entrance permit to the same places covered by the Golden Age Passport. The card will admit the holder and whoever else is in the car, or, if entrance is not by car, the holder and the holder's family. It also provides a 50 percent discount on all publicly run facilities and services.

There is also, for families, the Golden Eagle Passport, which costs $10, lasts the calendar year (January 1–December 31), and can be bought by mail or in person. It covers admission fees for the holder and family either in a private, noncommercial vehicle or on bikes or walking. It does not, however, offer any discount on services. Nonetheless, with entrance fees ranging from 50¢ to $3, it can be a money saver.

If you want to find out more about the passports, write to:
National Park Service
Room 1013
United States Department of the Interior
18th & C Streets
Washington, DC 20240

When is crying painful—and unnecessary?

When it's caused by dry eyes. But a new medication offers long-lasting relief.

More than a millon Americans—most of them women over sixty—suffer from this irritating problem, which is the result of an imbalance in the tear mechanism. They may have difficulty moving their eyelids, are sensitive to bright lights, and find it difficult to read. In many cases, the dry-eye condition, known as keratoconjunctivitis sicca, accompanies other problems such as arthritis, mumps, vitamin A deficiency, and thyroid disease associated with bulging eyes.

There are actually two systems of tearing. One is the constant flow of liquid that coats the eye with a film to keep the cornea moist. A second, backup system produces a large flow of tears in response to an emotional stimulus, to an irritant such as smoke or high wind, or even in response to a dry eye. Tears are composed of a combination of water, mucus, and fat. They also contain sugar, protein, and a bacteria-destroying enzyme that protects the eye against infection. When the balance of this system is thrown off, burning, itching, and a scratchy or sandy sensation may result.

Although the condition cannot be cured, it can usually be managed. The most common remedy is one of a wide variety of eyedrops available over-the-counter at pharmacies. It is important to consult your doctor before buying one at random, because the remedies correct different kinds of imbalances in the tearing mechanism. If you're also taking a tranquilizer, antihistamine, or decongestant, greater irritation can result.

For people who suffer from severe dry eyes, a new cellulose

123

tear replacement is now available. It melts in the eye, providing relief by keeping the eye moist for as long as twelve hours.

In winter, when the air is dry, humidifiers can also help relieve dry eyes. Air purifiers will help if the air is particularly dirty. Doctors recommend using white facial tissues, rather than colored ones, because the dye in colored tissues may irritate the eye.

Who says you don't have any rights in a hospital?

Whoever is telling you that is wrong. And with the cost of medical care what it is—nearing $300 billion annually in the United States alone—there's no reason to feel intimidated about exercising your rights.

Perhaps the most important right during your stay in a hospital revolves around the consent form. You have the legal right to be informed about and to consent, or not, to any surgery—and to restrict your consent to a given procedure. Your physician should explain what will happen in language you can understand and discuss it with you, answer your questions, tell you the risks. Don't be afraid to say no, or to ask, if you have any doubts at all, for a second opinion. And don't, preferably, get a second opinion from someone your doctor recommends; the collaborative effort between doctors often makes it difficult for a doctor to disagree with a colleague.

If surgery is recommended, ask about alternative procedures, about relative costs, about what the consequences would be if you chose to do nothing. Insist on seeing your medical records. Try to think of yourself as a partner in this with your doctor. Some doctors don't like this approach, but it's *your* body.

You should sign the consent form only after you're fully satisfied that the operation is necessary and you understand what it is and what its risks are.

Something else for you to consider if you're going to have an operation is the anesthesia. One of the reasons so many people stay in the hospital for so long after surgery is that they are recovering from the anesthesia. General anesthesia depresses the central nervous system, and slows circulation and the rate and depth of breathing. It's necessary in many operations—brain,

124

heart, and lung surgery are examples. But local anesthesia is used in a wide range of procedures, from childbirth to installing a pacemaker. Ask to see the anesthesiologist. Discuss the alternatives.

And before you even get to the hospital, you can help the treatment process by being sure your family doctor is ready to lend the hospital any of your records or X-rays that might be needed. (Don't forget information about allergies.) Members of your family can donate blood in your name. And for your purse's sake, double-check what will be covered by medical insurance.

What's in a bottle of booze that could be bad news?

Ever wake up the morning after with a headache even if you had only one drink? Or find that you've developed a rash? No, it isn't necessarily the alcohol, but it could very well be what's been added to it—like ethylenediaminetetraacetate, used to enhance the color in whiskey, or artificial flavors that create a "simulated cream base" in liqueurs.

If beer is your drink, the additives may range from acacia, a chemical to keep that foamy head intact, to the use of Yellow No. 5, a dye that can cause severe allergic reactions such as hives, sneezing, and asthma, especially in persons allergic to aspirin. If you prefer wine, your carafe could include malic acid to increase the vintage's acidity, or bentonite, a clay that clarifies the liquid, or hydrogen peroxide to remove the color from red and black grapes, or sawdust as a treating agent—and perhaps Yellow No. 5 too.

The trouble is you don't know what you're imbibing because at this time liquor, beer, and wine manufacturers don't have to list any of the scores of ingredients that are commonly used. Yellow No. 5, for example, must be specifically listed on all *foods* it's used in, but no mention is necessary when it's in an alcoholic beverage. Yet according to the U.S. Bureau of Alcohol, Tobacco and Firearms, there may be anywhere from nearly half a million to 1.7 million people who are allergic to the ingredients found in alcoholic drinks.

Regulations requiring a partial listing of ingredients were supposed to go into effect on January 1, 1982, but were squelched by the Reagan Administration. If you're interested in finding out more—and perhaps what your favorite libation includes (not all companies freely disclose what they put into their products)—a booklet, "Chemical Additives in Booze," is available for $4.95 from the Center for Science in the Public Interest, 1755 S Street NW, Washington, DC 20009. The organization has been trying since 1972 to get the federal government to require the listing of ingredients on alcoholic beverages.

Is aspirin a help or a hazard?

Overall, aspirin is a drug of long-proven value—but it does have some dangers, especially for pregnant women and children.

Considered by many to be as important a medicine as antibiotics, general anesthesia, and digitalis, aspirin has been used longer and more safely than any other drug. About 100,000 tons of it are produced worldwide each year.

In its yeoman role, aspirin is best known for combating pain, fever, and inflammation. And now aspirin has a relatively new lifesaving role in preventing heart attacks and strokes, by retarding the formation of clots inside blood vessels of the heart or brain. In the early 1970s, the Boston Collaborative Drug Surveillance Program found heart attacks to be less common among men who frequently took aspirin, compared with men who didn't. A British study found a 25 percent reduction in deaths among heart patients given aspirin daily for a year. And a Canadian study demonstrated that aspirin protected men who had suffered ministrokes from having later, more severe strokes.

Aspirin does its good deeds by blocking the synthesis within the body of prostaglandins, the hormonelike substances that induce fever, pain, and inflammation. It also blocks formation of thromboxane, a powerful blood-clotting agent, in platelets, the blood cells involved in clotting to stop bleeding.

This benefit for heart patients carries a peril for everyone else: Aspirin can cause slight bleeding from the lining of the stomach. This risk can be reduced by taking aspirin with milk, a glass of water, or food. Never drink alcohol at the same time; it can aggravate the bleeding.

Pregnant women should avoid aspirin because of its effect

on platelets, and because it might induce excessive bleeding in the mother and the baby in the first few days after birth. People with asthma are cautioned that it might cause a runny nose or bronchial distress. Aspirin may also actually make a common cold infection last longer—probably by inhibiting the body's production of interferon, which fights viruses. And, in combination with other drugs, aspirin can interfere with them or cause serious side effects. It can, for example, negate the effects of insulin.

There is now evidence—chiefly on the basis of studies by the National Institutes of Health—that fevers actually help the body fight off bacteria and viruses, and some doctors say moderate fevers should be allowed to run their course. Whether aspirin or acetaminophen should be taken if a fever is below 104 degrees is now being questioned.

A greater concern is that aspirin given to children when they have chickenpox or the flu may result in Reye's Syndrome (see page 44). In general, it should not be given to children unless care is taken against overdosing. As many as twelve thousand youngsters under five years old are treated yearly for aspirin poisoning; their bodies cannot absorb the doses that adults are accustomed to. For a child under three years old, give aspirin only as directed by a physician. At age three, one children's-size aspirin every four hours is the limit; from age four through five, two children's tablets. A child from age six through nine can take three tablets, and from ten through fourteen, four children's tablets, which are equal to one adult tablet.

The moral seems to be: When using a miracle drug, don't expect miracles unless you take some down-to-earth precautions.

What's a seven-letter word for a child who uses four-letter words?

H-e-a-l-t-h-y, according to child authorities, when the youngster is hurt or upset. Swearing releases tension, restores physical calm to the body, and provides a sense of control for children just as it does for adults. The trick is to get them to express themselves in other than "bathroom" language when in the presence of others.

Children are particularly prone to use "bad language" at two stages of development. The first is at nursery-school age, when they delight in using not only bathroom words but also sexual words whose meanings they usually don't know. The great up-surge occurs in early adolescence, chiefly as a way of showing how grown-up they are. Profanity, for example, gives boys a macho image and permits them to show interest in girls while at the same time keeping a distance emotionally.

If you're troubled by your child's swearing, experts advise:

☐ Focus on the feeling, not the words. What provoked your five-year-old to let loose a string of obscenities that would make a Marine drill instructor blush? Instead of saying "Don't use such language!" find out why the child is an-gry—and later point out that there are a lot of different ways to express anger besides using four-letter words.

☐ In an older child, redirect the desire to show off by, for example, improving the youth's vocabulary. Some teen-agers have found new and inventive ways to express themselves by using colorful language from Shakespeare.

☐ If you object to certain words, be firm about forbidding them, but don't overreact. When a young child uses words he or she doesn't know the meaning of, point out that they're not nice words and that you'd rather they weren't used. Offer to explain what the words mean if the child wants to know. Don't attach more importance to swearing than it warrants.

☐ Set an example and watch your own language. It's not really fair to expect your child to refrain if you let loose with "@#$%¢&*!" when you feel like it. Children don't pick up *all* their four-letter words at school.

Can roller skating be therapeutic?

Aside from being good exercise and good for the spirits, there's a chance that roller skating may also be good for pigeon-toes.

Little babies have cute little toes that turn in, but little chil-dren should have straight, forward-pointing feet with which to run and jump. There's nothing cute about the distortions to bones and posture, the clumsiness, and the price in self-esteem that pigeon-toes can cause. In severe cases, treatment may involve braces or even surgery. However, most problems, if caught in time, can be treated through exercise to correct the insufficient turning of the hip socket that produces the condition. Parents should make sure that the family doctor or pediatrician watches for signs of persistent pigeon-toes, especially if there is a family tendency in that direction.

Roller skating as therapy for pigeon-toes is the idea of Dr. Rosamund Kane, an orthopedic surgeon who directs the foot clinic at New York's Columbia Presbyterian Hospital. She thinks it makes sense because roller skating requires that the feet be straight. She cautions that parents check with the doctor before putting their toddler on wheels, because roller skating is effective only for certain types of toeing-in. But, she points out, a child who might not be conscientious about other exercises might be inclined to try harder when skating because it's fun. It's worth a twirl.

Do you have to be stuck with a lemon?

Not anymore you don't. If you bought a car that spends more time in the dealer's repair shop than in your garage, you don't have to grind your teeth about it.

In Connecticut, California, and New York, for example, it is the law that a dealer must replace your car or refund your money. In other states, about eleven thousand automobile dealers belong to the Automotive Consumer Action Program (AUTOCAP), an industry-sponsored arbitration system that handles disputes over malfunctioning new vehicles and has already earned a reputation of being fair and quick to decide. It's a good idea before you buy a car to find out if a dealer belongs to the program.

The common definition for a lemon is a car that has been in the shop for the same problem at least four times during the warranty period or within a year of the delivery date, or has been out of commission for at least thirty days in the same period. If your car fits that unhappy description, there are a number of ways for you to begin the arbitration process.

First, a number of manufacturers have their own arbitration mechanism. Others—General Motors, Nissan, Porsche-Audi, and

Volkswagen, for example—work through the National Consumer Arbitration Program of the Better Business Bureau. (Proceed by calling the nearest bureau office.)

Ford has its own arbitration panel, the Consumer Appeals Board, which is nationwide and has a toll-free hotline: (800) 241-8450. Its ruling is binding on Ford but not on the consumer.

Chrysler operates a Customer Satisfaction Board. Tell your dealer you want arbitration and you'll get a form to fill out to start the procedure. Chrysler's coverage, however, has earned a reputation for being restricted to certain items under the warranty.

American Motors and other imported cars except Mercedes-Benz handle their arbitration through AUTOCAP. If you want help or information, call (800) 555-1212 for the number appropriate to your location. Or you can write to AUTOCAP, 8400 Westpark Drive, McLean, VA 22102.

Shouldn't a stroke victim expect to be depressed?

Yes, of course, but there's a rub. Just because it seems normal for a person who has just had a stroke to feel depressed, doctors sometimes don't treat the depression. However, researchers at Johns Hopkins University School of Medicine have found that brain injury during stroke may cause not only paralysis but a depression as well—and unless the depression is treated, it may not go away.

While doctors have long known that depressions, some lasting for many months, may follow brain injury, there has been little effort up to now to treat them. One reason is that it's been taken for granted that disabilities as a result of a stroke would make anybody feel depressed. Another reason is that there has been little direct neurological evidence to indicate some particular abnormality that could be corrected.

The researchers, however, discovered in a study of 103 men and women who had had a stroke that depressive troubles were significantly more common among the patients with a stroke in the left half of the brain. These patients also had a high likelihood of developing depression within the first two years after their stroke. Many such depressions are severe and may at times lead to suicide attempts, the researchers said.

Depressive symptoms may also appear in chronically ill patients who had strokes ten or more years ago, particularly those with left-hemisphere brain injury.

If someone in your family suffers a stroke and depressive symptoms develop, don't assume they will go away on their own. Bring the patient in to the doctor. Treatment is possible with psychoactive drugs or other methods.

Should mother's milk always be on call?

Whenever you want it to be. According to the latest studies, breast-feeding on demand is okay.

Today's experts have reversed the counsel of yesteryear as the result of both new scientific evidence and observations of mothers and infants in so-called primitive societies. The experts now urge a return to a more "natural" pattern of infant feeding, including breast-feeding on demand.

Doctors used to think frequent nursing harmed the breasts, but a recent study reported in *American Journal of Diseases of Children* has shown that that's a myth. Researchers compared mothers who nursed on the usual three-to-four-hour schedule with those who nursed more frequently. The mothers in the latter group did not suffer from sore nipples more often than the other mothers. Nor did the frequent nursers experience more breast engorgement, that unpleasant, sometimes painful hardening of breasts that are too full of milk.

In addition, the frequent nursers had better supplies of milk. Surprisingly, however, the total time they spent breast-feeding was similar to that of the other mothers; they nursed more often, but the nursing sessions were shorter.

Short nursing times, an English study found, can provide adequate nutrition. Infants can satisfy their nutritional needs in only four minutes at each breast. They usually continue to suck for some minutes longer, but that may have nonnutritional benefits, such as strengthening the bond between mother and infant.

Also, newborns especially seem to need frequent feeding. It's been found that infants up to six weeks of age commonly seek to be fed every two and a half to three hours. Thereafter, the intervals between feedings grow longer.

The experts now advise a mother who breast-feeds to nurse her infant whenever she thinks the baby is hungry, and not to worry about overfeeding.

More and more of the experts are also urging new mothers to nurse their babies if at all possible, because evidence for the superiority of breast milk over cow's milk continues to mount. As the American Academy of Pediatrics says, breast milk is "the best food for every newborn infant." So let your baby have its fill.

Put my head in a paper bag? What for?

To prevent a migraine headache. British researchers tell of thwarting development of migraine attacks in patients by having them breathe in and out of a paper bag. This makes them re-breathe their own expired air, which is high in carbon dioxide, and that opens the restricted blood vessels that cause migraines.

The technique also frequently prevents expected migraine headaches from developing. Migraine victims sense, and show, signs of an impending attack, so the paper-bag treatment can be started when this warning or "aura" comes along.

As an example, researchers at London's St. Bartholomew's Hospital and the City of London Migraine Clinic cite a case involving a thirty-seven-year-old accountant who had had migraines since childhood. He had some usual symptoms—blind spots in vision and a drooping left eyelid—that ordinarily lasted forty minutes. They were followed by nausea and a headache lasting six hours. In an experiment, when an aura began, the man was told to rebreathe his own air in a paper bag. After twenty minutes he reported a slight headache, but no nausea. After another twenty minutes he said he was surprised to feel so much better so quickly.

In other patients, the rebreathing stopped twelve out of twenty-one attacks. The only side effect all the patients experienced was breathlessness.

Doctors aren't sure why this technique works, though they know that some migraine patients hyperventilate (overbreathe) during attacks. But they warn that breathing into a paper bag should be attempted only by migraine sufferers. Do *not* try it with other headaches. And discontinue the rebreathing if dizziness or lightheadedness occurs; too much carbon dioxide, or too little oxygen, can cause this unpleasant side effect.

When is a tummyache something more?

When it's IBD. An estimated 2 million Americans, including 200,000 children, have ulcerative colitis or Crohn's disease (ileitis), which are inflammatory diseases of the large and small intestines referred to collectively as inflammatory bowel disease, or IBD. Most people who have it ignore it—and that is neither wise nor pleasant.

IBD is not a tummyache that will go away. It is a chronic condition that requires proper diagnosis and treatment. Most people who have it can lead normal, active lives. Some, like President Dwight D. Eisenhower, can lead exceptional ones.

Doctors don't know what causes IBD, but it does tend to run in families, and scientists think that it may involve a malfunctioning in the immune defense system's handling of a viral or bacterial infection.

In addition to abdominal cramps, the symptoms include loose, bloody stool, diarrhea, and sometimes pain in the joints and skin sores. Crohn's disease can inflame the colon, rectum, anus, stomach, and ileum, which is the lower third of the small intestine. Other symptoms include fever and sores around the anus, as well as diarrhea and joint pains.

The treatment for both forms of IBD includes drugs such as sulfasalazine for mild cases, and corticosteroids such as prednisone for more severe ones. A good diet is especially important, because IBD is usually accompanied by loss of appetite and weight. Occasionally surgery is necessary to remove diseased sections of the bowel, but it's used only as a last resort.

Information, including special brochures for children and teenagers, can be obtained from the National Foundation for Ileitis and Colitis, Inc., 295 Madison Avenue, New York, NY 10017, (212) 685-3440, which has thirty-five local chapters across the country.

What's the latest news about the pill?

The latest news is mostly good. Researchers have decided that the pill confers a number of benefits aside from its chief one—providing the most effective contraception this side of celibacy. And they also think that women on the pill can do a lot themselves to reduce any risks.

Among the benefits, according to Dr. David A. Grimes of the Centers for Disease Control of the U.S. Department of Health and Human Services:

☐ Oral contraceptives appear to offer some protection against endometrial cancer, which is the most common cancer among women, and also against ovarian cancer, which is the most highly fatal.

☐ They also protect against benign breast disease and ovarian cysts. Although neither of these disorders is life-threatening, they are common, costly to diagnose and treat, and often require surgery.

☐ The pill also protects against other common gynecological ailments. It reduces by about half the risk of pelvic inflammatory disease, which accounts for at least a quarter million hospitalizations annually in the United States. Most women who take it also find that their menstrual pain lessens or vanishes altogether.

☐ Pill users' risk of ectopic pregnancy—pregnancy that occurs outside the womb, usually in a fallopian tube, and can be fatal—is lower than that of women who use other methods of contraception, and about one tenth the risk of women who use no contraception.

☐ Pill users appear to run less risk of developing rheumatoid arthritis than nonusers.

☐ Acne and oily skin improve among many young women on the pill.

☐ Reduced monthly bleeding decreases the risk of iron-deficiency anemia.

The risks of the pill have by no means disappeared, but encouraging new information indicates that users can take steps to reduce those risks. The most serious hazard is the risk of cardiovascular disease. Users are somewhat more likely than nonusers to die of pulmonary embolism, cerebral thrombosis, or myocardial infarction. However, the original studies showing this increase were done some years ago, when oral contraceptives contained much more estrogen than most of them do now. Scientists think today's pills probably cause only 1 or 2 cardiovascular deaths a year per 100,000 women under thirty who use them.

The women at highest risk are those with other risk factors: women with high blood pressure, high cholesterol, or diabetes, those over thirty-five, and, most important, those who smoke. Nearly 450 deaths in the United States every year are attributable to the pill's effects on heart and blood vessels—and could have been avoided if users hadn't smoked.

A woman on the pill can probably reduce her cardiovascular risk even further if, in addition to not smoking, she engages in aerobic exercises such as running or swimming regularly, at least twenty minutes three times weekly. Vigorous exercise helps by raising the blood levels of high-density lipoprotein (HDL), a substance present in the blood at high levels that is associated with reduced risk of coronary disease. Thorough workouts also increase the blood levels of plasminogen activator, a protein that helps break down blood clots. There's also the alternative, of course, of using another method of contraception.

Oral contraceptives can also interact with other medications. Scientists have discovered, for example, that pill users often react strongly to Valium. Researchers at Tufts University and New England Medical Center Hospital have found that even the small amounts of estrogen in the low-dose pills lengthened the time Valium remains in a woman's bloodstream by an average of thirty hours. Thus, women taking both medications may need to adjust their tranquilizer dose to avoid oversedation.

The pill appears to have no adverse effects on fertility after it is stopped, contrary to some early concerns. However, it may take women who have never been pregnant a few months longer to conceive than if they had been using a different contraceptive method. They may also stand a greater chance of having fraternal twins if they conceive shortly after stopping the pill.

Pill users do appear to get vaginal infections more often than nonusers, and perhaps urinary-tract infections as well, but many doctors think this may be traceable to increased sexual activity on the part of women who have been freed from worry about getting pregnant.

Well-known side effects, like nausea, fatigue, and other symptoms of early pregnancy, tend to be most noticeable during the first few cycles of pill use. Sometimes more serious symptoms appear too: high blood pressure, severe headache, and depression. Such symptoms should be discussed with a doctor.

Is "vagina" a dirty word for kids?

It shouldn't be. Child-development experts say an open attitude about sex with children will lead to healthier relationships when they're adults.

Sexual vocabulary—and, even more important, sexual attitudes—are strongly influenced by the vocabulary and attitudes children encounter at home. Yet even in a time when there is substantial public frankness about sexuality, most parents continue to find it tough to talk to their children about sex.

Researchers at the Project on Human Sexual Development in Cambridge, Massachusetts, caution that parental reticence about sex may have important impacts on a child's life. In addition to causing the youngster to be jittery about sex and sex talk, it could have related detrimental effects, such as making it difficult for a girl to use a diaphragm, or discouraging VD checkups and breast self-examination. Sexual misinformation can also lead, of course, to serious consequences such as an unwanted pregnancy.

Children as young as three are naturally curious about sex and reproduction—and will be exposed to sexuality in increasing ways as they grow older. Obviously, what a parent need tell a three-year-old will be simple and briefer than what a preteen is told—but the information, whether about menstruation, intercourse, or venereal disease, should be factual and made easy to understand. Use a medical-scientific term if necessary, but define it in a clear way.

Parents should also be aware that their own attitudes can unconsciously color the messages they convey to their youngster. Researchers at Florida State University at Tallahassee have found, for example, that when talking to sons parents emphasize the positive aspects of sex, but to daughters they stress the negative side. The small proportion of positive messages girls get from parents, the researchers noted, "are overlaid with negative messages that can produce ambivalence at best, and guilt and fear at worst. With this kind of ambivalence, it is not surprising that females express low satisfaction with their sexual experiences."

Experts also point out that parental messages about sex can be even more loaded if they come during the stress of adolescence. Yet because of their discomfort with the subject, parents often postpone discussions about sex until the teen years. That's usually a mistake. Anticipate the anxieties, doubts, and questions before they occur.

For the parent who would like to begin the discussion but doesn't quite know how to go about it, try using daily domestic events as a way to break the ice—a television program, a dinnertime conversation, or the behavior of friends, for example. And don't be afraid to call a sperm a sperm.

Double-jointedness—trick or trouble?

Don't wait for the pain to start to find out.

Double-jointed people perform tricks that the rest of us can't do. They can bend their thumbs to their wrists, or their fingers backward to parallel their forearms. They can touch the floor with the palms of their hands without the rigorous training dancers and athletes go through to achieve such flexibility. They can extend their elbows and the backs of their knees beyond a straight line.

Their friends call it a neat trick. Doctors call it joint laxity. It is observed mostly in youngsters, girls more often than boys, and for the most part it is not dangerous. At the least, however, it can lead to strain, because loose joints tend to be weak. In some instances, if it is accompanied by joint pain, stiffness, or swelling, it might be an indication of a joint or tissue disorder. One such disease is juvenile arthritis, which can be successfully and safely treated with anti-inflammatory drugs and physical therapy.

If you have a child who is double-jointed and who complains of pain or soreness in those joints, a thorough examination is your assurance that there is no underlying disease. The next step is to obtain from the doctor or a physical therapist a regimen of joint-strengthening exercises. For most people, fifteen minutes twice a day is enough to do the job. Swimming, walking, and skating are excellent conditioners. Other measures that may be suggested are special elastic bands, ankle weights, or arch supports for flat feet.

Body positions should be avoided that aggravate double-jointedness, such as sitting with crossed legs, Indian-style, or with a leg tucked underneath the buttocks. The knees should be slightly flexed when standing, never locked backward.

Double-jointedness can turn out to be a double whammy for children who suddenly find themselves demoted from prized performers of body stunts to "patients." They need to be reassured that they are normal, not disabled, and it may not hurt to suggest that a gorgeous backstroke or flashy figure-8 may be more glamorous than the tricks they used to show.

Are you ever too young to be depressed?

Unfortunately, no. Until recently many psychiatrists believed that children lacked the psychological development to experience depression. Not so. Most experts now agree that clinical depression is a real and widespread problem among children, even very young children. The National Institute of Mental Health estimates that one out of every five youngsters suffers its symptoms. And some psychiatrists believe that depression in the six-through-twelve-year age group may be massively underdiagnosed, because children often lack the verbal skills to express what they are going through and parents may not recognize the symptoms or may be unwilling to acknowledge them.

The primary symptoms of depression include loss of interest in normal pleasures and activities, poor appetite, sleeping disturbances, diminished ability to concentrate, lack of energy, a sense of hopelessness, and recurrent thoughts of death or suicide. Depressed children may be hyperactive or lethargic, or veer from one state to the other. They may exhibit hostility or overaggressiveness, may be reclusive, or have unusual difficulty with schoolwork. Teenagers may create excessive turmoil at home, turn to drugs or antisocial behavior, complain of psychosomatic aches and pains, and express low self-esteem and little interest in their future.

A child exhibiting four or more of these traits may be depressed. If the symptoms persist over weeks, it's a mistake for parents to assume it's just a phase. Depressed children often become depressed adolescents and adults. Suicide is the third highest cause of death among fifteen-to-twenty-four-year-olds.

Depression is often precipitated by a specific crisis, such as the death of a parent, separation, parental divorce, even a new baby. But it's still not well understood why some children (or adults) in these circumstances succumb to depression, as opposed to others who experience the normal cycle of grief and recovery. Sometimes there may not seem to be a clear-cut "cause."

There is growing evidence that both psychological and biological factors, including heredity, are involved. Dr. Joaquim Puig-Antich of Columbia University, who directs the child and adolescent depression clinic at the New York State Psychiatric Clinic, observed that in a group of depressed patients aged six to ten years old, the level of growth hormone in the blood was much higher than among normal children or among children diagnosed as neurotic but not depressed. He and his colleagues believe this finding can serve as a diagnostic test for depression.

Depression can be treated. Psychotherapy and, if necessary, a carefully monitored course of drugs can stabilize depressive patients and lift the pall of helplessness and hopelessness that characterizes their existence. The sooner treatment starts the better will be the child's chances of quick recovery without lasting scars. Many medical centers now have adolescent-care units. Advice can also be sought at the unit, from pediatricians, or from a local county medical board.

Does your teenager avoid the eye doctor because he's afraid he'll have to wear specs?

Well, tell him there's a good chance he may not, even if he's complaining about things getting fuzzy while studying. The problem may be a case of muscle fatigue, and that may benefit from eye-muscle exercises that can be taught by an ophthalmologist, an optometrist, or an orthoptist, an eye doctor who specializes in the treatment of ocular muscles. Once learned, the exercises can be done at home.

Many vision problems have to do with eye muscle balance, such as convergence insufficiency, or the inability to turn both eyes toward the nose adequately when looking at a close object. In some cases eyeglasses may not correct that.

If you're the one with the problem, there is a chance that you can be helped, too. There can be many reasons for blurred vision and you should first have a thorough examination by an eye doctor. If there is no medical disease of the body or refractive error requiring glasses, eye muscle exercises may be of help.

If you think you or your teenager has an eye problem produced by a muscle imbalance, here are two tests you can try:

To check convergence, look at the tip of a pencil at arm's length. Slowly bend your arm to bring the tip toward your nose. If the pencil appears to double before it's within four inches, you may have a convergence problem. To improve it, repeat the test as an exercise for five minutes every day. If after a month the problem has not gotten better, see an eye doctor.

To test the eye's ability to focus, stand twenty feet from a wall with a picture on it. (If you wear glasses, you can put them on for this exercise.) Hold a book at arm's length. Look at the picture for a few seconds, then look back at the book, then back to the picture again. If you have trouble focusing from one to the other, practice this, too, as an exercise, and as you get better at it, bring the book closer to your eyes and shift your focus more rapidly. If after practice you still can't do it, you might need glasses or a new prescription.

There is also an exercise for tired eyes. If you or your child has a great deal of close work to do, stop every twenty minutes and look into the distance for sixty seconds. Focusing at long distances keeps the eyes parallel and allows relaxation of the muscle effort required to focus on near objects.

Are there other uses for a waterbed?

Yes, indeed. Waterbeds are being used in hundreds of hospitals all over the world as healing aids.

Doctors have found that waterbeds distribute the weight of patients more evenly than other kinds of beds, and they've begun to use them increasingly in the treatment of certain patients. For example, waterbeds reduce both bedsores and skin and tissue breakdown, a particular and often fatal problem for severely paralyzed and paraplegic patients.

French doctors have found that gently pulsating water mattresses placed in the incubators of very premature babies have reduced both apnea (interrupted breathing) and bradycardia (slowed heartbeat), both of which are causes of crib death. Researchers at Stanford University and the University of Colorado also discovered that premature babies placed on waterbeds tend to eat better and to gain weight more quickly than preemies on regular mattresses. Presumably, the stimulation and relative weightlessness created by the pulsating waterbed simulate the in-utero environment.

Waterbeds, heated to at least 80° F, have also been used successfully to treat both arthritis and lower back problems. A recent study published in the *Journal of the American Society of Psychosomatic Dentistry and Medicine* showed that waterbeds enabled insomniacs to sleep and regular sleepers to sleep longer and feel better throughout the day. And a waterbed makes it more possible for a pregnant woman to sleep on her stomach.

Waterbeds cost about the same as regular beds. If your doctor prescribes one, it can be tax-deductible. So if you have a sleeping problem, maybe it'll float away.

Do dental braces have to hide a smile?

Not anymore. Now the smile can hide the braces.

Lots of adults need to have their teeth straightened for cosmetic or health reasons. The American Association of Orthodontists estimates that one out of every four current orthodontic patients in the country—some 800,000 people—is over eighteen. But now there's the chance of wearing braces without anyone but the dentist knowing.

Invisible braces are the invention of Dr. Craven Kurz of Beverly Hills, California. He calls them lingual appliances, because they fit on the tongue side of the mouth, behind the teeth. In addition to being hidden, Dr. Kurz's braces are easier to clean and more comfortable than conventional ones, although somewhat more complicated to install. The period of treatment is about the same, from eighteen to thirty months, but the cost is about a third higher.

Since their introduction in 1982, over a thousand orthodontists have learned how to fit lingual braces. During this time, Dr. Kurz and a group of other leading practitioners have monitored the new method and have continued to work toward making it as effective as possible. At present, however, they do not recommend lingual braces for anyone with extremely short or small teeth.

For people who need or prefer conventional-style braces, there are other innovations such as clear or white plastic ones. There's also a new type of brace that is being used alone or in conjunction with traditional braces—a plastic mouthpiece known as Occlus-o-Guide, worn for only part of the day. It's recommended for children whose permanent teeth are still coming in. Treatment with the mouthpiece has been running from $400 to $600.

A good bite is critical to the health of teeth and gums. Although braces are expensive, they are much cheaper in the long run than gum surgery and false teeth. Most orthodontists will work out a plan for installment payment, and some dental-insurance plans cover part of the cost. So if you need braces, at least you can now grin and not bare it.

What are the ifs, whens, and buts of sitting?

No buts about it. If you spend lots of time sitting, make sure you have the proper chair. And when sitting, keep moving.

The United States today is a sitting society. White-collar employees outnumber blue-collar workers by 20 million, according to U.S. Census statistics, and more than half our working hours, it's estimated, are spent sitting—to commute to work, at work, during coffee breaks, at meals, in front of the TV set.

Unfortunately, many people don't have the proper chairs for all that inactivity, and the wrong chair is as bad for you as a pair of shoes that don't fit. Experts estimate that workers perched on ill-designed chairs lose an average of forty minutes of productive time each day.

Sitting long stretches is bad for your health anyway. Gravity leads fluid to collect in the ankles and feet, causing swelling, or pedal edema. Being in the wrong chair only compounds the problem. Among the physical ailments associated with poorly chosen chairs are backache, headache, fatigue, insomnia, and impaired blood circulation.

In choosing the correct chair, experts say you should check for four factors:

1. Make sure that the chair's height keeps your hip joints and your knee joints flexed at right angles and your feet flat on the floor. That's a fancy way of saying sit up straight.

2. The backrest should fit snugly in the small of your back to support the lower spine.

3. The seat should slant slightly backward to allow you to lean against the backrest. Its edge should not dig into the backs of your legs. Also, if you have to turn a lot to reach different equipment or to complete tasks, be sure the seat swivels so that your entire torso can move as a unit.

4. The material covering the seat should be porous, to allow body heat to escape. No vinyl.

Proper chair or no, physiologists advise that you not stay seated for long. When traveling, get out of your car, plane, or train seat every hour or so and walk around. In the office, get up from behind your desk every so often for a stroll. Pace while on the telephone. At the very least put your feet up on the desk now and then to avoid swelling in the ankles and feet.

Keep moving even when you're sitting down. Do leg spreads, walk and run in place, cross your arms, do side bends.

And if you have to stay seated, mimic your children, fitness experts advise. Squirm, kick your legs up and rotate your ankles, swing your arms and clasp your legs to your chest, roll your head around on your neck. It's one healthy activity kids seem to have come by naturally.

Can you calm the chronic go-getter?

Yes, the behavior of the "Type A" personality can be modified—so much so that the risk of a second heart attack may be reduced in men who undergo behavior training after their first attack.

The intense, self-driven person, usually a man, was first

dubbed a "Type A" personality, highly susceptible to heart attacks, by Drs. Meyer Friedman and Ray H. Rosenman of San Francisco. Subsequently, a blue-ribbon panel convened by the National Heart, Lung and Blood Institute "solidly established" Type A as a heart-attack risk factor along with cigarette smoking and high-fat diets.

Dr. Friedman heads a five-year Heart Institute study of about a thousand heart-attack victims to see what effect will come from calming them down. So far, about 60 percent of the men have changed their behavior, and their chances of having a second—and fatal—heart attack seem to be reduced.

Type A personalities can be recognized by their tendency to be quick to anger, tense, hard-driving, and impatient. They are likelier to have elevated blood pressure. Some make heavy use of personal pronouns—"I," "me," "mine." They think of doing two things at once, hurry the speech of other people, and make a fetish of always being on time. Even with children they play nearly every game to win, and have difficulty just sitting still.

As part of a calm-down treatment, Type A's are urged to "drive in the slow lane," to eat slowly, to speak slowly, to listen to the conversation of others. They are advised to stay away from violent programs on TV, and to spend at least twenty minutes each day in quiet time, both mentally and physically.

Physical exercise helps, too. At the Duke University Medical Center, researchers put men and women, aged twenty-five to sixty-one—all of them the rushed, aggressive, driven Type A's—on a ten-week program of stretching exercises, vigorous walking, and jogging. And down came Type A behavior.

If you think you're a Type A, try the restraints and exercises yourself. Or meditation. They're all a do-it-yourself opportunity for better health—and a longer life.

Is it any wonder you can't remember anything?

Maybe you don't have any "wonder."

Memory is crucial to every aspect of our lives, but all of us experience times when memory fails us, often embarrassingly. And some people claim they can never remember a name or a face.

Although the psychological and physiological bases of memory formation and retrieval are only beginning to be understood, researchers are learning some fascinating things that can help us remember better. For example, wonder.

Common sense tells us we remember best what we're interested in. Junior draws a blank with French verbs but remembers every big-league pitcher of the past twenty years. Now research is confirming the power of curiosity. In several studies where subjects were shown faces and asked to frame questions—"Would I buy a used car from this man?" "Is she an actress?" "Is that person shy?"—they remembered faces better later than when they used standard memory techniques such as noting a person's hair color or head shape.

The opposite side of the coin is stress. Just as children often don't learn well when they're frightened, habitually stressed people can be too distracted to form clear impressions. In the same way, it's hard, when under stress, to get in touch with the deep parts of the brain where memory is stored, which is why relaxation techniques such as meditation and hypnosis are great aids to memory.

When you're nervous and upset, the last thing you want to hear is someone telling you to relax. However, you can learn techniques that will improve your memory. Some are used by those memory marvels like Harry Lorayne, who make their living showing off fantastic feats of memory.

When meeting a stranger, in addition to noting facial features and asking yourself questions such as whether you'd buy a used car from that person, make name-picture associations. If you meet a man named Green, try to visualize his face as green. If it's a harder name, ask for the spelling and see the letters in your mind. Repeat the name in conversation (with the images in your head), and especially as you say good-bye.

If you have a number of errands to run, rehearse the sequence of them mentally. See yourself getting into the car, stopping at the bank, etc. That way, even if you forget to take your list, you may not forget what's on it. And make your lists in categories of things or events, no more than seven categories or seven items per category. Seven is what psychologists say is the maximum cluster we can retain.

Create your own mnemonic devices (from Mnemosyne, the Greek goddess of memory). They can be rhymes ("Thirty days hath September . . ."), sentences from initials ("Every good boy does fine," the EGBDF treble notes of the G clef taught musical students), or pun associations (we "spring forward" or "fall back" when setting clocks for standard or daylight-saving time).

If you're studying for an exam or memorizing a speech, do it in the evening. It's been found that long-term memory works better as the day goes on, and sleep will help block interference from other memories. In addition, study in time chunks of twenty minutes, if possible, or of no more than two hours, if you're really pressed, before stopping to refresh, rest, and review.

Don't worry that your memory is failing because you're getting older. Clinical senile dementia is rare. But brains, like bodies, need exercise. Memory may slow up a bit with age—doesn't everything?—but it is not lost.

There is a new body of research that suggests that certain foods rich in the chemical choline, such as eggs, soybeans, and liver, may help the brain chemistry of memory. Whether or not this is so, there is no question that proper diet and exercise are essential to all good brain and body functions. And what is definitely known is that alcohol impairs memory.

Now that genes can talk, what can they tell us?

How to be healthier and have healthier children.

Genes are the chemicals on the chromosomes in our cells that determine our heredity. but in addition to Mom's red hair and Grandpa's nose we can also inherit a tendency toward a specific disease.

Some genetic disorders are largely concentrated in particular racial or ethnic groups—sickle cell anemia among blacks, beta-thalassemia among people of Mediterranean origin, Tay-Sachs disease in Jews of Eastern European background. Some disorders—such as a tendency to diabetes or early heart disease—run in families.

As medical science learns more about genetic disease, more and more people are being helped through genetic counseling to minimize health risks and to cope with real or potential problems. Perhaps most important is the help now available to potential parents who know or suspect they may carry the genes of disease.

146

There are now about a hundred genetic diseases that can be detected prenatally. These include Down's syndrome, Tay-Sachs disease, and the neural tube defects that cause severe brain and spine deformities. Among the tests used is amniocentesis, in which a small amount of the amniotic fluid the fetus floats in is removed from the womb. Analysis of the fluid can determine the fetus's chromosomal makeup.

When grave problems are found, a couple can decide whether to have the child and how best to care for it. In the vast majority of cases, however, the happy result of prenatal testing is to provide the joy and reassurance that they may look forward to a normal baby. In fact, several reports show that genetic counseling and prenatal diagnosis encourage childbearing. One report from Boston University, based on a survey of seventy-seven genetic counseling centers, showed that the number of counseled couples planning to have children was 14 percent higher than the number of uncounseled risk-aware couples. A British study found that such help greatly eased the concerns of beta-thalassemia carriers and was coupled with a significant reduction in abortion rates.

In addition, in what is considered a major breakthrough, scientists at the National Institutes of Health and the University of Illinois College of Medicine recently succeeded in altering the activity of genes in patients suffering from thalassemia. As reported in the *New England Journal of Medicine,* the scientists were also able to improve the blood chemistry of sickle cell patients. The result, based on the use of a drug called 5 Azacytidine, are considered preliminary but hold great promise for future treatment of anemic disorders.

Information on genetic counseling can be obtained from the National Genetics Foundation, 555 West 57th Street, New York, NY 10019; from the National Foundation—March of Dimes, 1275 Mamaroneck Avenue, White Plains, NY 10605; or from organizations concerned with particular diseases.

Is there a "time of the month" for sex?

For sex, no. For sexiness, likely.

Human beings have the capacity for sex anytime, unlike other animals which couple only when the female is in estrus (heat).

But *when* we want sex, or want it most, may be influenced by the same factors that regulate estrus in other species.

The female menstrual cycle and other reproduction-related functions are regulated by hormones. Female hormones are called estrogens, male ones androgens. But each sex has some of the other's hormones, though not in as great quantities. The level of estrogens in a woman's blood peaks at the time of ovulation, which corresponds to estrus, the time when an egg can be fertilized. Not surprisingly, there is a correlation of heightened sexual feelings in women at this time of the month, and it's been assumed that estrogens were responsible, but apparently it's not as simple as that.

A number of studies, most recently a joint investigation by researchers at the University of Pennsylvania and Downstate Medical Center of the State University of New York, have shown that it may well be a woman's level of testosterone, the principal male hormone, that's the key factor, if not the only one, in a greater sexual drive. Testosterone and desire levels were found high in women not only at ovulation, when estrogen is high, but also shortly before and after menstruation, when estrogen is low. Both these times are often periods of heightened sexual desire, too.

A subtle interplay of hormonal factors were also found: A woman can be influenced by the level of her partner's testosterone, and *his* testosterone level may be heightened by pheromones produced by her higher hormone level. Pheromones are sexual scent signals. The human signals may be more subtle than those of other animals, but they're there.

Although studies of the effect of hormones on sex drive, as well as on mood, are still in an early stage, what's clear already is that there probably are times when "yes" can be expected and times when "no" is not a rejection but a biological phase of the month.

Are you getting all the nutrients you need?

In our health-mad society, it's ironic that so many of us are not. A new study by the Department of Agriculture reveals that many Americans are lacking in six vital nutrients—vitamins A, B_6, and C, calcium, iron, and magnesium. Half of us don't consume enough B_6, one third don't get sufficient vitamin A, one fourth are short on vitamin C. Iron intake is below recommended levels for 82 percent of all infants between one and two years old and for about 70 percent of women twelve to fifty years old.

To assure yourself an adequate diet, eat a variety of foods daily that includes fruits, vegetables, whole-grain and enriched breads, cereals, and grain products, milk, and cheese. But avoid fats. This can be done by eating lean meat, fish, poultry, and dry beans and peas as your protein sources. Also, broil or bake your food rather than fry it. Limit your intake of butter and shortening, and stay away from too many eggs and organ meats such as liver.

Eat food with adequate starch and fiber (carbohydrates). Carbohydrates have an advantage over fats because they contain less than half the number of calories per ounce. Complex carbohydrates—such as beans, peas, nuts, seeds, fruits and vegetables, and whole-grain breads—are better than simple carbohydrates—such as sugar—because they contain many essential nutrients in addition to calories.

Read the labels on the food products you buy so that you know exactly what you're eating. If you feel you're not getting enough vitamins, consult your doctor before adding a vitamin supplement to your diet.

Is there hope for the anorexic girl?

Indeed, yes. But working out of the problem isn't easy, because it is a self-induced condition, largely psychological.

The ailment is known as anorexia nervosa, a self-inflicted starvation, stemming from obsessive fear of becoming overweight, that can be fatal. It mainly affects girls, with one estimate that 1 out of every 250 girls between the ages of sixteen and eighteen is an anorexic. (Only 1 boy is for every 30 females.)

Among the techniques that have been developed to resolve the problem is Nurturant Authoritative Psychotherapy. In it, the therapist or counselor takes a direct approach, telling the self-starving youth how to act, what school classes to take, what to eat, how to direct behavior so as to eventually restore self-esteem. It is said to be effective in more than eight out of ten cases, but early treatment is important.

The youngsters most often afflicted with anorexia are teenage girls from middle- and upper-class families. Often such a girl is the "model child" in a family that puts a high value on achievement and appearance. She usually weighs at least 25 percent less than ideal weight for her age and size, but insists she's fat, and may suffer certain other physical signs: lack or cessation of menstruation, a skeletal look, sandpaperlike skin, low blood pressure, downy hair on body and face, facial puffiness, even an orange-yellow skin color.

Sufferers from anorexia nervosa often become emaciated, but don't seem to care. Some binge on food, then make themselves throw it up. There can be a variety of precipitating factors. The anorexia may be brought on by some emotional crisis, or by fear of becoming sexually mature. Some girls, convinced they are nobodies, dull and uninteresting, believe it is the only way to draw attention to themselves. Many are budding ballerinas, continually concerned about weight and height and trying to forestall development of a full, feminine body.

Besides limiting herself to a few hundred calories a day, the anorexic may abuse laxatives and diuretics, or overexercise in an attempt to burn up calories. The victims usually deny they have any problem, and so don't seek help. Parents and friends come to despair.

For further information about Nurturant Authoritative Psychotherapy or further understanding of this complex problem, contact the National Association of Anorexia Nervosa and Associated Disorders, Box 271, Highland Park, IL 60035.

When should you start caring for your baby's teeth?

Nine months *before* the baby is due. Recent studies have demonstrated that if you take fluoride tablets during pregnancy, your child will have fewer cavities—a fact well known to Australian obstetricians, who have prescribed them for tens of thousands of their patients over the last twenty-five years. And it's considered safe for the baby.

The studies also found that fluoride tablets taken during pregnancy may have other helpful effects besides preventing cavities in almost every child whose mother took them. These women seemed to bear fewer premature babies, and the babies were larger. There is even a hint that fewer birth defects occurred in this group.

Although baby teeth usually don't erupt until some months after birth, they actually begin forming in the fetus before a woman reaches the fourth month of pregnancy. Even some permanent teeth begin forming around the sixth month.

You should start taking fluoride tablets when you're three months pregnant, even if you live in a community with fluoridated water and use a fluoride toothpaste. Those sources don't provide enough fluoride to ensure that your baby's teeth will be so strong and smooth that decay can't get started. So when your doctor confirms your hunch that a new family member is on the way, ask for a prescription for fluoride tablets.

Take the tablets on an empty stomach, and don't consume milk, antacids, or supplements containing calcium immediately afterward. And every time you take the fluoride, give yourself a pat on the back for sparing your unborn child painful hours later in the dentist's chair—and for sparing the family bank account, too.

What's a bigger trauma than divorce for a youngster?

Remarriage. It at once strikes the deathblow to a child's fantasies of his or her parents' reconciling and forces the youngster to forge a relationship with an unknown person who can exert control over what the child does.

There are now stepchildren in one out of every four families, and more children are entering such families every day as divorce and remarriage occur with greater frequency. "These 'reconstituted,' 'combined,' 'blended,' or 'step' families have significant and difficult tasks to master as they attempt a life together," says Elinor Rosenberg of the Department of Psychiatry at the University of Michigan Medical Center in Ann Arbor. "Children continue to mourn the loss of the original family, struggle with loyalty conflicts and sexual tensions with unrelated family members."

The trauma of a remarriage may be intense for youngsters. A recent study of 742 school-age children found that those living with stepparents were more likely to show signs of depression than were those living with their natural parents or with a single, divorced, or separated parent. The distress emerges in many ways: tension or arguments with the new stepparent or sibling or even the natural parent; forgetting school assignments or skipping classes; rebelling against curfews, bedtime, or doing daily chores.

Some of the trouble may be avoided, child experts say, if new couples are especially sensitive to the children right from the time of their wedding, even though that is when they are savoring their own relationship. The experts advise keeping disruptions in the children's lives to a minimum. For example, don't rearrange all the furniture. Keep the usual dinner hour and serve familiar foods. Save romantic candlelit suppers for when the children are in bed or away.

When trouble occurs, don't hesitate to call on the ex-spouse for help. "People who don't feel that they have to continue a vendetta can use one another in an intelligent, friendly way," says Dr. Clifford Sager, head of the Remarried Consultation Service of the Jewish Board of Family and Children's Services in New York City, and clinical professor of psychiatry at New York Hospital–Cornell Medical Center. Grandparents, on both sides, and aunts and uncles may also be able to help relieve some of the strain. Dr. Sager's tips for new stepparents:

- ☐ Don't try to make the stepchild into your own child by acting the role of the biological mother or father.
- ☐ Do express your views about the child's behavior. The home the child lives in is your home too. But let your mate do the disciplining until you've established a trusting relationship with the child.
- ☐ Don't expect your stepchild to love you from the start. Have patience. Give the relationship time to develop.

In a crisis, the family can turn to counseling. Mental-health professionals can often help resolve conflicts through psychotherapy. Your state mental-health association can provide information.

Though remarriage can cause some problems, it can also be a rewarding experience for youngsters. "If the situation is well handled," says Dr. Sager, who has four stepchildren of his own, "the child has a wider range of models for himself—which can be extremely enriching."

How do you frighten off the bogeyman?

By exposing him for the fraud that he is—and helping your child understand what a nightmare means and how normal it is to have one.

A nightmare is a way a child tells "in pictures" something he or she cannot express in words—a fear about school, jealousy toward a sibling, anger at a parent. And you, the parent, can help.

- ☐ Be calm. If you're upset, the child will be too. Reassurance and comfort are needed.
- ☐ Don't kill the monster, shoot the bear, or lock the witch in the closet. Tell the child there is no monster under the bed, in the chair, in the closet. A child's capacity for differentiating between fantasy and reality is shaky, and you don't want to perpetuate the difficulty. There are no such things as monsters, so they can't "go away." They don't exist—period.
- ☐ Be sure, however, that the child understands that you understand that the nightmare was real, even if the bogeyman isn't. Don't make light of it.
- ☐ Talk about it. Ask how big the bad thing was, what color, how close it came. Don't be afraid that recalling these things will revive the fear. Talking the dream out, experts agree, helps to dispel its effect. And don't be surprised or hurt if the monster begins to take on a striking resemblance to you. Parents are figures of power and therefore of fear as well as of love and protection. (It has been suggested that family dream-telling sessions, around the breakfast table, for example, help a young child to realize that others also experience nightmares.)
- ☐ Put on a night-light or the radio and leave the door ajar when you say good night again.

If bad dreams recur frequently, they may indicate psychic trouble. When persistent nightmares follow a traumatic event—such as severe illness, a death in the family, or parental separation—psychiatric help may be advisable. But for most children, nightmares shouldn't automatically be thought of as a sign of trouble. Contrary to a long-held assumption, children's dreams are not deeply symbolic and complex, according to Dr. David Foulkes of Emory University, who directs the Cognition Research Laboratory of the Georgia Mental Health Institute. He believes, as the result of studies of children in sleep laboratories, that their dreams are simple and reflect the limited events of their own lives and intellectual capacities. Pediatric psychologist Carolyn Schroeder, for example, recalls a significant rise in the number of children's nightmares reported to her at the time the film *Star Wars* was first released.

The moral: Fear is a nightmare your child can understand and conquer.

When is martyrdom not saintly?

When it's marital martyrdom—the widespread habit of suffering in silence when a spouse does something upsetting. For example, a woman may resent it if her husband spends the weekend watching sports on television, but she resolves to say nothing. Or a man may expect his wife to initiate sex, and hide his disappointment if she fails to do so.

Unfortunately, unlike the saintly kind of martyrs, marital martyrs usually try to get even. They find some way to make the spouse feel guilty, or they save up their resentments until they finally explode. On the other hand, they often seem to need their martyrdom, and find it hard to give up.

Of course, lots of annoying personal habits ought to be ignored. Marriage counselors point out that since no two people will agree on everything, a certain amount of live-and-let-live is necessary in any relationship, especially one as intimate as marriage. But true marital martyrs don't simply let their spouse's annoying behaviors slide by: They bite their tongues, but nurse a grudge.

If you feel resentful about something, ask yourself whether it's really important. If not, resolve to put it out of your mind. If that's not possible, reflect on what your spouse's behavior may mean to you on a deeper level. A woman who thinks she's mad at her husband for not taking out the garbage may really be angry about his more general failure to do his share in running the household—a common source of tension today, when the majority of wives work outside the home.

Most important, if you decide your complaint is important and legitimate, don't suffer in silence. Speak up. Remember that no matter how close you are, your partner can't read your mind. You may be surprised at how willing a spouse is to try to change once it's clear that something's really bothering you.

When you do speak up, observing a few simple rules can help resolve the situation without creating ill will on either side—and give you a better chance of achieving the changes you want:

☐ Pick your time and place carefully. A spouse who's just had a run-in with an important client is obviously not in a frame of mind to be reasonable about a complaint from you.

☐ State your gripe calmly and without anger. You're trying to start a discussion, not a fight.

☐ Instead of being accusatory, describe your complaint in terms of your own feelings. Not "You never take out the garbage!" Instead, "It upsets me when you don't take out the garbage."

☐ Recognize that your spouse has complaints about you, too. If your criticism prompts one in return, the two of you may be able to negotiate a verbal contract in which each of you agrees to work harder to change a behavior that upsets the other one.

Maybe neither of you will be able to change a habit that's troubling, but you'll at least be laying the groundwork for an honest and lasting relationship.

Can canker sores be avoided?

If you're lucky, you've never even wondered. Some people get them, some people don't. No one knows why for certain, but recent research indicates that canker sores may result from injury to the soft tissue of the mouth in those who are susceptible. By avoiding injury it may be possible to avoid the recurrence of those nasty little ulcers that doctors call aphthous stomatitis. Whatever they're called, they can make for a miserable week or two.

In a study conducted at the National Institute of Dental Research, thirty patients who had suffered from canker sores over periods ranging from five to fifty-five years were tested along with fifteen volunteers who had never had them. After local anesthesia was administered, small puncture wounds were made in their mouths. Of the susceptible group, thirteen developed canker sores. None of the controls did.

The troublemakers in daily life that might be responsible include hard-bristle toothbrushes, toothpicks, sharp utensils, and hard or sharp-edged foods like peanut brittle. Nuts seem to be a prime offender, but whether as a result of biting down hard on them or because of possible allergy is unclear. Too vigorous dental flossing can cause minor cuts, too. The National Institute researchers also suggest that deficiencies in iron, vitamin B_{12}, or folic acid may lead to injured tissue.

A healthy diet and tender loving dental care are the best means currently advised for preventing canker sores.

Who's the safest person on the job, in the home, on the road?

Someone over sixty-five. He or she has a lower accident rate than a person under sixty-five, whether at work, at home, or in a car. According to a recent study by the National Center for Health Statistics, the accident rate for people sixty-five years old or older is less than two thirds that of younger people.

Statistics show that although the slower reaction time of older people results in their producing less, their work and the quality of their output are more consistent than their colleagues', and their accident rate is lower.

Seniors tend to adjust to their slowing reaction time and their diminishing visual perception in the automobile, too. It's true that they drive less often, but when they do their accident rate is about the same as that of middle-aged drivers and lower than that of drivers under thirty. So if Grandmother or Grandfather wants to drive and has no serious vision, hearing, or health problem, relax.

156

No matter how good their safety record, it's still wise to take a few precautions in the home to avoid injuries that can prove serious to older people:

- [ ] Never wax floors to a slippery high gloss.
- [ ] Leave a 25-watt light bulb on at night.
- [ ] Mark the "on" and "off" settings on the stove with clear writing, perhaps on tape with a red marker.
- [ ] If certain items are used frequently, leave them on easily reached shelves.
- [ ] Attach grab bars to the wall of the tub and the wall near the toilet, and provide handrails on the stairways.
- [ ] Paint the bottom and top steps in contrast to the other steps, or put a bright strip of tape on the carpet of the bottom and top steps if they're carpeted. Most elderly people who fall on the stairs fall on the last step up or the last step down.
- [ ] Keep thresholds to less than ¼ inch high to avoid tripping.
- [ ] Never rearrange the furniture without telling the seniors in the house. When you do rearrange it, don't put anything in the middle of the room or in a travel path.
- [ ] Be sure the seniors in your home know the exit paths in case of fire. Check with your fire department—some have stickers to identify seniors' windows.

When should life be all play?

In infancy and early childhood. Many child psychologists are now discouraging educational toys and "lesson games" and urging parents and nursery schools to shift their emphasis away from planned activities, which the experts believe are turning play into work. Play, they insist, should be playful. And, they point out, young children never forget what they learn for themselves—as opposed to what they're taught.

Play actually begins at birth, with mouth play. An infant moving his or her tongue around the nipple after being fed or blowing bubbles with saliva is playing. Infants as young as a week old enjoy imitating those around them, too—sticking out their tongues or wiggling their fingers in response to an adult who does so.

Babies begin playing with their own bodies, especially their hands and feet, as they grow a little older and begin to get control of their muscles. But even when they're a month old and can't reach out for objects, they "play" with their eyes, staring wide-eyed at anything that interests them.

From about six months on, babies love it if you make faces at them. And face-making is valuable, too. At this age babies become fearful of strangers, and when familiar people make funny faces it helps babies be less anxious about strange new faces in their world.

Although cooperative play with other children doesn't begin much before the age of three, children are interested in each other long before that. Psychologists now think that babies actually begin trying to play with other children around the age of one. But at this age playmates tend to treat each other as objects, not people—which is why toddlers playing together have to be watched carefully to prevent hair-pulling and toy-snatching.

What can you do to encourage a child's play? Focus on the interests of your youngster, not your own. Provide freedom for children's imaginations. But set limits, too; it's possible to overstimulate children. And once you've started a child on an activity, let the youngster carry on alone.

Vigorous play, including vigorous outdoor play, is important, many experts believe, but so are daydreaming and pretending. Encourage both kinds. Life should be all play for the first few years.

Can money grow on trees?

Yes, indeed—shade trees. The money comes in the form of hefty savings on your fuel and utility bills.

Many people don't realize that a few carefully selected trees strategically placed outside a house can significantly reduce heating bills in the winter and cooling costs in the summer.

About a third of home heat can be lost as cold air moves in through openings around doors and windows and other gaps. That loss can be as much as two thirds on a day when there's a stiff fifteen-mile-an-hour breeze. Planting a row of evergreens as a windbreak on the windward side of the house can reduce heating costs by as much as 20 percent. The trees pay for themselves in fuel savings in just a few years.

Planting deciduous trees—which lose their leaves every fall—on the east, west, and south sides of the house can both cool it in the summer and warm it in the winter. In hot weather, the trees screen windows from the sun and create shade on the walls and roof. Moreover, because they draw water from the ground and evaporate it through their leaves, they can cool the air around the house by as much as fifteen degrees. In a fully shaded house, air conditioners work only half as hard as they do in an unshaded one—an obvious saving. After they lose their leaves, deciduous trees help warm a house in cold weather by letting the sunshine in.

When you decide to sell your house, shade trees can also help you get more money for it. Government studies show that attractive shade trees in the yard can increase a house's market value by as much as 15 percent.

Furthermore, trees provide noneconomic benefits as well. They help clean the air we breathe by trapping dust particles. And a four-foot-wide row of trees around your house will dampen neighborhood noises. Besides, they're beautiful.

When can lying on your left side cure a disease?

When you're expecting a baby and have developed toxemia—or, as it's more correctly called, pregnancy-induced hypertension.

The condition, which occurs in 5 to 7 percent of expectant women, develops late in pregnancy, usually after the twenty-eighth week. The characteristic signs are a sudden and excessive gain in weight, swelling of the face, hands, and feet, protein in the urine, and elevated blood pressure. In severe cases, there may also be persistent headaches, blurred vision, and dizziness. The disease can progress to include convulsions. Toxemia is the third leading cause of death among pregnant women in the United States. It also is a serious threat to the well-being of the child.

No one knows what causes the disease. Doctors once thought—incorrectly, it turns out—that the fetus produced a poi-

159

son that entered the woman's bloodstream; thus the term "toxemia." Today scientists believe that the condition occurs because the woman's circulatory system fails to adjust to the increased demands of the pregnancy. The disease usually disappears shortly after the baby is born.

Certain groups of women seem more susceptible to developing pregnancy-induced hypertension. They include women expecting their first child or those carrying twins, teenagers, women over thirty-five years old, those who are either underweight or obese, and women who have diabetes, kidney disease, or high blood pressure to begin with. The condition recurs in a quarter to a third of women in subsequent pregnancies.

The key to managing toxemia is early detection. The goal is to check its progress so as to ensure the woman's health and to permit the baby to mature to term and be safely delivered. With that in mind, doctors recommend regular prenatal visits to monitor the condition of both the woman and the baby.

Women at high risk of developing toxemia are urged to eat a well-balanced diet rich in protein. Once pregnancy-induced hypertension is diagnosed, the prescription is plenty of bed rest. Usually that is enough to stabilize the condition and retard its progress. Women who find it impossible to stay off their feet at home—because of the demands of toddlers, for example—are sometimes hospitalized to ensure complete rest. Doctors recommend that women lie on their left side, not on their backs. The position permits maximum blood flow to the uterus and the kidneys by relieving compression of major blood vessels caused by the pregnancy.

If you have any of the warning signs of toxemia, call your obstetrician immediately.

What's better, sleeping on the job or taking a coffee break?

A short snooze, say sleep experts, if you're a natural napper.

The fabled afternoon siesta has a rotten reputation as the refuge of the lazy and weak-willed, but the reputation is undeserved. Napping is actually normal, healthy behavior, a natural response to human body rhythms that society has suppressed in all except babies and the elderly. President Harry S. Truman was a well-known napper. John F. Kennedy, too.

A short sleep break can dissipate stress, increase alertness, and even boost productivity. As researchers at the University of Pennsylvania found, people were better able to solve mathematical problems after a brief rest.

Naps are probably the ideal solution to the doldrums that hit nearly everyone each day about midafternoon. Much better than a coffee break, in fact. The stimulating caffeine in coffee works against the body's natural rhythmic peaks and ebbs in energy. The snooze need not be a long one; fifteen minutes of shut-eye is as refreshing to many people as two hours is to others.

But naps, it should be noted, are not for everyone. Roughly half the population, for as yet mysterious reasons, are just not able to take forty winks. And they should not. When they do, they have a tendency to get up groggy and irritable—and unable to sleep at night. But if you have the ability and opportunity to nap, take advantage of it. It's a natural talent.

When does retirement mean going to work?

Increasingly, older Americans are returning to work, either reentering the labor force on a part-time basis or volunteering their time and expertise. And government and business are making it easier for them to do so. The result: The retirees are living longer and are healthier.

As of 1983, the federal government lowered the age at which senior citizens can return to work without losing their Social Security benefits, from seventy-two to seventy. Also, there's a growing need for workers as the birthrate declines. Furthermore, the myth that old age necessarily brings with it infirmity and senility is beginning to be exploded. Corporations are finding that older workers are more committed, and more skilled, than younger workers.

Flexitime and flexiwork are two concepts being put to work for retirees. Instead of hiring one person full time for a job, some companies are using two or three people part time, or combining functions of several jobs and dividing them among several people. In one successful program, the Travelers Corporation, an insurance company in Hartford, Connecticut, created three hundred shared jobs for six hundred retired employees.

Many businesses are also allowing retirees to work up to 120 full workdays without losing their pension. This way they can hold a full-time part-time job. Other corporations get around pension problems by contracting the work to outside agencies and then recommending their retirees to those agencies.

For further information, write:

Association of Part Time Professionals
Post Office Box 3635
Alexandria, VA 22302

National Council on Aging
600 Maryland Avenue SW
Washington, DC 20024
(For $3.50, it will send you a booklet, "Part Time Employment after Retirement.")

If you don't want to return to work but still want to be useful, you can join the more than 4½ million older Americans doing volunteer work. According to the Retired Senior Volunteer Program, a federal program that has placed over 250,000 retired men and women in jobs, volunteers are working in organizations that couldn't otherwise afford them, solving housing problems, and providing income and nutrition counseling, among other things. They're working in hospitals, correctional facilities, nursing homes, museums. Some have joined the Peace Corps. And many of them say that in exchange they're keeping young.

For more information, check your phone book under "United States Government Offices" for your regional ACTION office, or call toll-free (800) 424-8580.

Instead of throwing in the towel when you reach seventy, toss in your hat and keep active. You'll thrive in many ways.

Are young lovers friendly?

To each other, yes. To others, no—and they couldn't care less.

If those wedding bells are breaking up that old gang of yours, don't be offended. It's normal. Social scientists, not as poetic as songwriters, call the phenomenon "dyadic withdrawal" from the "interpersonal network." ("Dyad" being a fancy way to say "couple.") Sigmund Freud put it more simply: "The more two people are in love, the more they suffice for each other."

However you describe it, it seems that most young lovers go through a period when they lose interest in their friends. According to a study of dating couples at Pennsylvania State University, a process of withdrawal takes place that becomes more and more selective as the love relationship intensifies. Peripheral friends go first, but there is also a clear decline in the importance of the companionship or opinions of even previously "best" friends. This is equally true for males and females.

Does it happen because it's "natural," something biologically determined? Or because our culture expects it, giving out signals that lovers are supposed to live only for each other and be left alone? The experts disagree. In the Penn State study, many couples reported a *greater* involvement than before with relatives, and a deeper concern for their opinions. Society seems to provide, through family, the rituals for keeping young lovers, moonstruck though they may be, within the social order.

Is it nepotism to bring your kids into your office?

Not if they're six years old.

If you worked on a farm or lived over the store, as many shopkeepers used to, your family—even the youngest members of it—would see you at your job. But if you work in an office, you may not have thought to have your children visit you there. You may think it's inappropriate or that they wouldn't understand what you do. You may not even talk about your work with them at home.

By denying your children knowledge of what you do and the chance to see where and how you do it, you're cutting them off from a major part of your life. You're also preventing them from learning that the world of work is part of their lives, too, as members of a family and as people who will also work one day. As one guidance expert points out, many children now grow up with little understanding of what work is, and what adult skills are.

A parent's job is something that should be shared with children. It should be explained as much as possible, including the problems. Children who have had a crotchety teacher are capable of relating to your woes with a difficult boss. Knowing that you're having a rough time at the office can help children cope when you're frazzled and blue. (And they will be less likely to assume that they're responsible for your bad mood.) When things go well, they can share in your pleasure and sense of accomplishment.

They should also understand why you work. As one teacher expressed it, many children seem to understand money only as something to be spent, with no awareness that it is also something that must be earned.

A visit to your office can help make work a concrete reality for your children. They may not fully grasp the significance of a purchase order or a claim form, and you may have rough going to make clear exactly what an account executive does, but even very young children can appreciate that the activity around them is serious and that you play an important role in this hustle-bustle.

Introduce them to your fellow workers. Talk about what you're doing as you do it. If you're afraid they may become restless and misbehave, plan some things they can do to help you—"real work," like stuffing envelopes or pasting stamps.

When children can actually visualize where you are and what you're doing during the day, they are more likely to feel secure in your absence and more positive about it. Nowadays, when many mothers as well as fathers are breadwinners, work should be a family affair.

What can you do to help your child overcome shyness?

Don't mention the word—ever, at all!

Research shows that two out of every five children are shy, some perhaps predisposed to it from birth. But although the blushing and trembling associated with shyness are embarrassing, they can be overcome. It's a question of building up your child's sense of self-esteem, according to psychologist Dr. Philip G. Zimbardo and Shirley L. Radl of Stanford University.

First and most importantly, never call your child "shy." Considerable research supports the theory that labeling becomes a self-fulfilling prophecy. If you call your child "shy," the child may believe it and become even shyer.

Secondly, expose your child to as many people of all sizes

and ages as you can. Invite other children over to play, and take your child frequently to the park or playground. Or join a play group, the Brownies, or the Cub Scouts. And don't be afraid to leave your child in the care of another adult. Children who never leave their parents tend to be shyer than others.

To build a sense of security, hold, touch, and cuddle the youngster. Talk to your child and listen to the answers. Teach the youngster basic social communications—"Hello," "How are you," "Thank you," and "You're welcome."

Also, encourage your child to take risks and be adventurous. Working puzzles, learning arts and crafts, learning how to tie shoelaces, etc.—all help to build self-confidence.

And it's very important, too, not to be disappointed in a youngster. Develop realistic expectations of what your child can and cannot do. Putting too much pressure on a child or showing disappointment can also cause shyness.

Above all, don't you be shy about showing your love and understanding. That's a happy antidote to the problem.

What can you do to prevent your teenager from smoking?

For one thing, forget about those traditional warnings—how he or she may develop cancer or heart disease thirty to forty years from now. That's an awful long time away for a teenager to contemplate.

Instead, point up the immediate consequences—the bad breath, smelly hair, yellowing teeth, and a much-less-than-perfect performance on the athletic field. That, researchers say, works.

Peer pressure plays an extremely important role in the decision to start and to continue smoking. And to stop smoking, too. In a model program involving eight thousand seventh-graders in the Minneapolis area, nearly half of those who smoked broke the habit. They did so after attending small discussion groups led by someone their own age, not a teacher.

By the way, the seventh grade—when a youngster is on the verge of adolescence—is the most effective time for such discussions. Most young smokers—chiefly boys at this age—have not yet developed an addiction to nicotine, and only 7 to 10 percent are "regular" smokers—that is, one cigarette a week. By the ninth grade, girl smokers outnumber boy smokers.

One thing the discussions include is how to say no to the offer of a butt without being ostracized. The answers are practiced in scenes acted out by the youngsters. At the end of a five-session program, students are asked to pledge not to become regular smokers. (The use of the word "regular" permits the freedom to experiment.) The pledge session is videotaped and played back to the entire class.

According to the researchers who did the study for the Laboratory for Physiological Hygiene of the University of Minnesota's School of Public Health, a follow-up on 1,500 students in a pilot program found smoking levels cut in half among those who had participated in the smoking discussions. Data from two later studies involving 3,200 students showed a 75 percent reduction in the habit.

As for those who think chewing tobacco is an alternative to smoking, the negative also prevails. Doctors say that chewing the weed can destroy gums, lead to the loss of teeth, even contribute to causing cancers of the mouth. Tell the kid chewing is unsightly, smelly, and—because you have to do something with the spittle—socially a downer.

What's in your kitchen that roaches would die for?

Your own chemical-free zappers, which could be just as effective against certain pests as regular pesticides.

Crushed cucumber skins and bay leaves are particularly effective against roaches, according to experiments performed by Professor Clifton Meloan of Kansas State University in Manhattan, Kansas. He put them in a tank with some sixty cockroaches, and it turned out that, in the laboratory at least, the cucumber skins and bay leaves drove the roaches away.

During the course of his experiments, Meloan isolated the most active roach-repellent compounds—cineole in the bay leaves and cis-6-trans-2-noneal in the cucumber skins. Try spreading that combination around daily wherever you have a roach problem. Or try boric acid, also an effective cockroach-repellent poison.

You can also make some homemade sprays to fight plant bugs. One of the most effective on both indoor and outdoor plants is an onion-and-garlic mixture. In the blender mix four cloves of garlic with one large onion and two teaspoons of red pepper (cayenne or chili) or two finely chopped fresh hot peppers. Blend the mixture with two cups of water for one minute in the blender. Let it steep overnight. The next morning, strain it through a worn pair of pantyhose or some cheesecloth, add a tablespoon of detergent, which will help it stay on the plants, and dilute with five cups of water. Then use the mixture once a week until the bugs are gone.

An effective home remedy for spider mites is a spray made of two tablespoons of buttermilk mixed with one cup of flour and diluted with one gallon of water. This, too, you should use once a week until the mites disappear.

Soap and water mixed together have proved a scourge for aphids, mites, mealybugs, lacebugs, and scales, when they're young and their shells haven't yet toughened. As soon as you see any, mix one tablespoon of mild soapflakes per gallon of water and use once a week until the problem is solved.

Many home pesticide recipes are based on the theory that a plant that is susceptible to or already afflicted with bugs can be successfully rid of bugs if sprayed with concoctions made from plants that are immune. Chives are the most famous of these. To make "chive tea," chop up chive leaves and combine with boiling water, in the ratio of one teaspoon of chopped leaves to one cup of water. Let steep for fifteen minutes, strain, and then spray.

Finally, if you can stand it, you can collect dead bugs and make a bug-juice spray from the very bugs that are giving you the trouble. Blend them with two cups of water and spray them on the plants under attack. Then sterilize the blender!

Does your child want a nose job?

Think twice before agreeing to it—or to any operation involving plastic surgery. Surgery before full growth has ceased can be detrimental, causing psychological and social difficulties.

According to Dr. Melvin Spira, head of the Division of Plastic Surgery at Baylor College of Medicine in Houston, more and more teenagers are seeing plastic surgeons about having operations for a variety of deformities or what they believe are disfigurements. One particular group includes teenage girls as young as fifteen years old. So embarrassed by large breasts that they avoid athletics and won't wear a bathing suit at the beach, they seek breast-reduction operations. Others, boys and girls, want their noses reshaped, or their protruding ears flattened. Still others hope to do away with acne.

All these operations, as well as those to correct birth defects such as cleft palate, are possible. So, too, are operations to redress deformities and burns that result from accidents. But the question, says Dr. Spira, is whether they should be attempted. For one thing, is it the parent who is pressuring for the operation? For another, is the patient a depressed individual who is seeking plastic surgery to relieve the depression? No responsible plastic surgeon wants to operate on such a person.

Be aware that a patient is not always satisfied. Major scarring can sometimes result, depending on an individual's skin type and the way incisions heal.

Whether for a child or an adult, if you're considering plastic surgery the choice of physician is absolutely critical. Many quacks abound, so be sure that your surgeon is fully qualified—that is, certified by the American Board of Plastic Surgery, or an ear, nose, and throat specialist experienced in handling ear and nose surgery. Be wary of such phrases as "Board-certified cosmetic surgeons" or "Cosmetic surgeons certified in their specialty," many of whom are too willing to operate without considering all the implications involved.

Plastic surgery can do a great deal of good, radically altering a person's self-image in a positive way. But its success depends on the person, the degree of deformity, and the age at which it's undergone.

Is working part time really good for high-school students?

Maybe not. For some youths, a job is a necessity, a way to help out at home or save up for college; for most others it's simply a way to earn some extra pocket money. Recent studies show that a part-time job can be an important earning and learning experience for teenagers—but it can have undesirable effects as well.

American youngsters have always worked, but today a greater percentage of teenagers juggle work and school than at any time in the past twenty-five years—about half of all high-school juniors and seniors and almost a third of all ninth- and tenth-graders. They are also working longer hours than the high-school students of yesteryear.

The good news is, first of all, that working teenagers enjoy the feelings of productivity, satisfaction, and confidence that accompany a paycheck. Though most of them work primarily to earn spending money, they still contribute indirectly to family finances by freeing funds that might otherwise have gone for clothes and an allowance, or the expenses of running a second car. Furthermore, they earn parental respect doing so.

Their spending is important to the economy, too. Researchers at the University of California at Irvine, who conducted a large-scale, government-funded study of the costs and benefits of part-time employment in high school, found that the hundreds of students in their study earned, on average, more than $200 a month. And they generally work at low-paying jobs without fringe benefits, not in competition with adult job seekers.

Working is valuable for noneconomic reasons, also—to learn practical lessons about how the business world operates and how to manage money. Working teenagers are forced to organize their time, to be responsible, and to learn to get along with others in the workplace.

Now for the bad news. Working leaves teenagers less time to spend with their families and friends. In addition, most jobs available to teenagers are boring and unchallenging. Few of them teach skills that will be useful later in the adult work world. Furthermore, many teenagers spend their hard-earned money on alcohol, marijuana, and other drugs.

The most important detrimental effect, however, is on grades and on attitudes toward school. Many students—especially borderline and poor students—develop a distaste for school after they've begun to work, and their grades suffer.

The number of hours worked, of course, greatly influences school performance. The University of California study disclosed that tenth-graders seemed to be able to work up to fourteen hours a week without damaging their grades, and eleventh graders managed up to twenty hours with no apparent ill effects.

Should your teenager work? If it's not an utter necessity, be a clock watcher regarding the hours involved and monitor school performance closely. There are times when the lessons to be learned by working are of less importance than a youth's school and family life.

How do you deal with the temper tantrums of the terrible twos?

Ignore them. Child-behavior authorities agree that, though it's hard to do, pretending indifference is the most effective way to calm down that howling, head-banging, blue-in-the-face terror, a toddler in the throes of a full-scale temper tantrum.

Once you understand why tantrums get started, it's easy to see why this is sensible advice. Imagine that you are in a foreign country but don't speak the language. All around you people are talking—to each other and to you—but you can't respond, or even ask basic questions. Pretty frustrating, right? You want to scream. That's exactly how toddlers feel when they're beginning to learn how to talk. They understand language but have not yet mastered it enough to convey their desires and make their own comments on the world around them. The result: extreme frustration, which can turn quickly into rage.

Not all children are tantrum throwers, but among those who are, tantrums usually begin just before the age of two and tend to be at their worst between the ages of two and three. Children outgrow their inability to talk, of course, and their frustration at being unable to communicate vanishes as they get more verbal. Whether they outgrow their temper tantrums as well depends a lot on how you react to them.

Suppose you respond, as your instincts may tell you, by giving the child your complete attention, by making frantic efforts to quiet the youngster, by fulfilling the child's desires. You're doing what behavioral psychologists call reinforcing the temper tantrum: You're teaching the child that throwing a fit gets him or her what he or she wants. There are better ways.

The temper-tantrum habit should be nipped in the bud, advises Virginia E. Pomeranz, associate clinical professor of pediatrics, Cornell University Medical College, who offers several tips to make a household tantrum-free. First, you can do a lot to keep a tantrum from ever getting started if you're alert to a child's state of mind and sensitive to the youngster's boiling point—and yours. Tired, hungry children are vulnerable to tantrums. If a meal is going to be delayed, a snack may be in order. A child who's had a taxing day can profit from a warm, soothing bath before dinner. Don't let your own taxing day make you too quick to respond with a sharp "No!" to any harmless request the youngster makes.

If the storm does explode, don't lose your cool and act panicky. Awful as that breath holding looks, the child will not be hurt. Don't lose your temper, either; appear tranquil, and don't express anger in any way. Pick the child up, tell him or her calmly that this is not acceptable behavior, and take the youngster to a room to be alone—preferably his or her own room. Explain that the child will stay there until he or she feels better—and stick by what you say.

"The 'punishment'—deprivation of attention—is entirely appropriate," Pomeranz says, "and you have conveyed an important message: nice behavior is rewarded by the opportunity for social interaction; nasty behavior results in just the opposite. The message will get through."

Should there be sex after a mastectomy?

Why not? According to Dr. Mildred Hope Witkin of Cornell University Medical College, a mastectomy in no way impairs the physiological functioning of sex. In fact, many women report that their sex life actually improves after the operation. And it in no way alters the sexual response for most men.

Myths abound, however, about mastectomies. Among the most common is the feeling of being "half a woman" and of being repugnant to a male partner. Actually, the vast majority of men don't leave the mastectomy patient. In fact, the husband or lover usually becomes more considerate and affectionate.

Another myth is that the mastectomy wound and the resulting scars will be repulsive to a man. One of the best ways of coping with this fear is to encourage the man to be present in the hospital when the dressings are changed. The quicker reality is faced, the quicker the adjustment to it. To ignore the situation—to treat the woman as though nothing has happened—can be psychologically damaging. The woman then cannot unburden herself of her feelings, and her repression can delay recovery.

A mastectomy, like all major operations, is a traumatic experience. The woman's body is altered, and a new body image must be built up. Emotional swings and periods of depression often follow the operation while this new image is developing.

One helpful way to speed up the process is to resume sexual activity as soon as possible after the operation. In fact, Dr. Witkin suggests that sex be tried the first or second day after the woman arrives home from the hospital, not necessarily to experience orgasm but to help the patient recognize that she is still sexually desirable. If husbands fear they'll seem unfeeling or too demanding if they express a desire for sex this soon, they should realize the enormous emotional boost their partners will probably experience.

Love and communication are the basic ingredients in a good relationship, and when these are present, the absence, size, or shape of breasts becomes unimportant. The trauma and the brush with mortality often bring couples closer together. The shared experience can result in an increase in the frequency and variety of their sexual activities, and an even more satisfactory sex life can be attained.

Is sex bad for high blood pressure?

To the contrary: It can be healthy even for people with hypertension, as high blood pressure is called medically. Intercourse does boost blood pressure somewhat, but only momentarily. It doesn't affect the underlying basis of hypertension.

Orgasm usually produces relaxation, a release of nervous and muscular tension. Avoiding sex because of fear that it might affect you adversely doesn't make sense, because sexual activity has no connection with the mechanisms that cause elevated blood pressure.

Some drugs prescribed to control hypertension may, however, also curb the sex drive and even make some men impotent. This side effect can often be handled by reducing the dosage of the drug, or by switching to a different drug. The new drug will, hopefully, be as effective against the hypertension but have less potential effect on the sexual mechanism.

A medication that causes impotence should never be simply abandoned without being replaced. To do so could be dangerous. A patient should insist on a full and frank discussion about possible side effects with his doctor.

Sexual dysfunction can adversely affect the overall health of a patient. So sexual counseling is a vital adjunct in treating the high-blood-pressure sufferer.

How do you tell if your teenager drinks?

First of all, do you drink? Studies show that 81 percent of the time, if both parents drink, their children will, too. Conversely, 72 percent of parents who abstain have children who abstain.

Most teenagers, especially boys, start drinking at the age of thirteen or fourteen. For some it is an expression of normal, adaptive behavior and an introduction to adulthood. Often they join their parents in having wine or beer at the dinner table without ill effect. These teenagers drink infrequently and consume only small amounts of wine, beer, or liquor.

However, according to the National Institute on Alcohol Abuse and Alcoholism, some 450,000 people under the age of twenty-one are already alcoholics. The teenagers in this group usually drink with companions, rather than at home, as a way of expressing rebellion and independence. They drink less regularly than older people but consume a larger amount of liquor on a drinking occasion. Unfortunately, having acquired little tolerance for alcohol, many teenagers become daring and impulsive under its influence. If they drive while intoxicated, the result can be fatal.

Teenage alcoholics tend to share with adult alcoholics feelings of isolation and the need to have a drink to calm shaky nerves. They exhibit aggressive behavior toward family and friends, and frequently express grandiose feelings of superiority and omnipotence. Inside, however, like all alcoholics, the teenagers feel guilt, remorse, and despair. They also become uncomfortable in situations where there is no alcohol, and are continually preoccupied with wondering when they can have the next drink. This causes loss of interest in outside activities and an attitude of not caring about other people.

Are you worried that your teenager is an alcoholic? Sometimes the evidence is clear. Does he or she continue drinking when others have stopped? Drink more frequently and consume more? Seem to have an increasing tolerance for liquor? Have early-morning tremors? Drink in the morning? Lie about his or her drinking?

Teenage drinking is also characterized by falling grades at school and a sudden decrease in penmanship skills. The young alcoholic is likely to be absent or tardy at school, and not have a long attention span. Also, he or she is giddy and giggly, impulsive and rebellious.

Helping teenage alcoholics is difficult because frequently they will not discuss the problem. If, for example, you think your son is an alcoholic, confront him, but do it in such a way that you establish your love and show your concern over the change in his behavior. Point out these changes to him, and don't be afraid to seek professional help.

Alcoholics Anonymous offers assistance, as do other groups, including churches. If you need advice and guidance, ask your minister or rabbi, or check the phone book for a local AA chapter.

Will he always prefer a young chick?

No. That's a myth that usually accompanies the myth that all men go through a mid-life crisis.

It is not unusual for a man to go through a period of critical self-examination at the age of forty, forty-five, or fifty. But that doesn't mean he will perforce decide he has failed in life or that life has failed him, that time is running out, that a young woman will, if not rejuvenate him, at least make him feel younger for a while.

Several long-term studies of men suggest that an inability to adapt to change, poor self-image, damaged self-esteem, and unexamined depression, anger, or fear can all precipitate a full-blown mid-life crisis. But that doesn't happen to each and every man.

What does occur is that most men (and women) reassess their lives as they reach the forties. Where am I? What have I accomplished? What do I have left to do? What would I like to do? These and other questions are perfectly natural and, indeed, a healthy step in the transition to middle age. Often they lead to a change in environment, to a new job or occupation, for example, or to moving to a different part of the country.

The man who does chase youth is a man with problems— and needs counseling. But researchers find that he's in the minority and that too much has been made of the problems of middle age. Rather than a step toward the end, Carl Jung, the famous psychologist, had a better term for it—the "noon of life."

Is your health a private matter?

It should be, but unless you're careful about what you sign and with whom you sign, the answer is "no."

Many life-insurance companies, including many of the largest, require you to sign a "medical authorization" before they will consider your application—a mere formality, if you believe most salespersons, who often fail to explain what it is and what its implications are.

When you sign a medical authorization you give your doctor permission to give out your complete medical file to the insurance company through a data bank called the Medical Information Bureau, which holds the files of more than 11 million people in the United States and Canada. It holds them for several years.

Companies subscribing to the bureau have access to whatever is in your file simply by asking for it and paying a minimal fee. They use the information as a basis for deciding whether you qualify for medical or life insurance. Included in your file can be information relating to anything from heart disease to suicide attempts.

Although few people are told this, the information on file may be given, without permission, to member companies of the insurance firm.

The bureau's rules state that subscribing members *must not* use its reports as the sole ground upon which to judge a life- or health-insurance application. But in 1977 a Federal Trade Commission investigation found that some companies were doing just that and other companies were using the bureau files to check on job applicants.

If you are interested in protecting your privacy, if you want a personal health evaluation for an insurance application that will be confidential, apply for insurance with a company that doesn't subscribe to the Medical Information Bureau. There are more than a thousand of them. Question your sales representative.

If you have already signed a medical authorization, you have the right to request your file from the bureau. However, although companies can get the file directly, an individual cannot. The file is sent instead to your doctor (who, by the way, is not legally required to show it to you). If the doctor lets you see it and it turns out that the file contains inaccuracies, you can correct them without charge.

To write for your file, send your name, birth date, and birthplace to Medical Information Bureau, P.O. Box 105, Essex Station, Boston, MA 02112. The bureau will send you form D-2, a disclosing form in which you absolve the bureau of any responsibility that might result from use of your file. Many consumers object to signing this, but without doing so they are unable to proceed further. When the bureau receives the signed form, it sends your file to your doctor, who may share the information at his or her discretion.

How can you be picky about a pediatrician?

First of all, select yours in advance. When choosing a pediatrician, or an internist, or a cardiologist—whatever kind of doctor you seek—it takes time to get the information you need to pick the right one, but it is time well spent. All doctors are not alike. The differences in their training, specialties, hospital affiliation, and even personalities can have significant bearing on the health care that you and your family receive.

Primary-care doctors, as the name implies, are the ones you need first and usually most. They are the doctors who check you out and can treat the normal range of illness and injury: the family doctor, who is generally an internist, a specialist in internal-organ medicine; the pediatrician, for the children; a gynecologist, for the females in the family. Doctors trained in family practice cover all these areas, and for people living in remote places they are often the only nearby primary medical resource.

Where choice does exist, it can be confounding. Most people begin by asking friends, relatives, or co-workers, which is a good way to learn at least how promptly appointments are kept and how congenial your informant finds the doctor. Knowing a doctor's age and sex is important in making a personality match, and should be part of your considerations. A person who, for example, finds it difficult to talk about intimate problems with a doctor who is much younger or of the opposite sex runs a serious risk of jeopardizing his or her health.

You can also get referrals from the medical department of your company, if one exists, from the medical society in your community, or from a local hospital. The last should be a university-affiliated hospital, if possible, because they are usually more selective in their staff, and doctors with teaching responsibilities tend to be more in touch with what's new in medical treatment.

You can check the qualifications of the recommended doctors in the *Directory of Medical Specialists*, available at most public libraries and at medical libraries. Where doctors have done their internships and residencies is more important than where they went to medical school. Again, the university-owned or -affiliated hospital is best. The doctors on your list should ideally be associated with such a hospital, if there is one in your community. It can affect the care you receive from other specialists, such as anesthesiologists, radiologists, and the like, if you are ever hospitalized. These hospitals also tend to have more up-to-date equipment. A study by the Stanford University Center for Health Care Research shows that a patient's chance of dying or suffering serious complications following surgery can be two and a half times greater at a poorly run hospital.

Having made a few preliminary choices, you should not hesitate to find out about what these doctors charge for office visits and checkups. Where you don't get the information clearly and cheerfully, cross that doctor off your list. If a doctor's nurse is rude or inefficient, remember that you're going to have to deal with that go-between every time you need the doctor, and how quickly you can get your message through in an emergency may be critical someday.

When you finally make an appointment for a checkup, be

sure you note how thoroughly the doctor takes your family and medical history, how carefully you are listened to, how well the recommended tests and procedures are explained, how clean the office and equipment are, how new the medical books and periodicals around are, and whether you feel rushed or relaxed. If these all check out, you've got yourself a doctor.

If the time should come that you need a specialist, your primary-care doctor will probably refer you to one or two. If time permits, you should check their qualifications with the same care you used for your family doctor. And by all means, get more than one opinion if a course of treatment is involved that you are in any way concerned about. If surgery is needed, play the numbers. The more operations a surgeon has performed in his or her specialty (assuming they have been successful, of course), the safer you will be. Be persistent in asking for such information.

A doctor is a human being who happens to be trained to give a specific and very important service. If you are not afraid to check the competence and qualifications of an auto mechanic but you are scared to ask about a doctor, your car may be in better shape than you are.

Is bigger better?

Yes, if you're a basketball player. For the rest of us, it is—or should be—unimportant.

Pygmies in Africa are superb elephant hunters, but they do it by stealth and brains, not brawn. Yet the prevalent attitude, particularly marked in Americans, is that bigger is better. It's a point of view that can be devastating for short people, of whom there are an estimated 7 million in this country.

Short people, children and adults, are often patronized or taken less seriously than their taller counterparts. It's annoying when you're ignored in a busy store. It's enraging when you're passed over for promotion in favor of someone taller (hence "maturer"). Short women have to fight the image of cuteness, short men of being considered unmanly.

It's understandable that a young child responds well to being thought of as a "big girl" or "big boy," because a child's job is to grow up in size and skill. But it's not wise for too much emphasis to be put on size alone. Comparing heights among children, and praising the youngster who grows faster, makes no sense either. Many children are slow to develop, and some are never going to be tall; stature is largely a matter of genes, unless there is a problem of malnutrition.

One pitfall parents face is being too overprotective of a small child out of fear that he or she might not be able to cope with school or play situations. Similarly, some parents expect tall children to behave older than their age, and that can be damaging, too.

Height problems intensify in adolescence. The very short boy or very tall girl wonders if he or she will be socially and sexually acceptable. Some sensitive teenagers simply withdraw from social interaction or take up inappropriate behavior, perhaps clowning too much or habitually making fun of themselves (before others can).

The single most important factor in the development of a healthy attitude toward height is the parent who can instill respect for human diversity, pointing out the great number of achieving short people—Mickey Rooney is a good example—and of the varieties of activities in which height is not important—tennis, swimming, music, for example.

Parents who brag about their son's height, columnist Ann Landers once pointed out, may not have anything else they can crow over.

Want to dream your troubles away?

You can and you do—naturally. With training, you might be able to do it even better.

Dream researchers are learning that dreams do seem to help people cope with problems and that we tend to dream more when under stress. One such expert, Rosalind D. Cartwright, chairman of the department of psychology at Rush Presbyterian–St. Luke's Medical Center in Chicago, notes growing evidence that "we can train ourselves to have conscious control over our dreams." Working with recently divorced women, she found that some of them were able to change the plots of repetitive, distressing dreams related to their failed marriages, incorporating instead more optimistic endings. In another study she directed, she found that patients who worked at retrieving and discussing dreams had a higher rate of success with subsequent psychotherapy.

Gayle Delaney, a San Francisco psychologist who specializes in dreams, has a system that she claims helps her patients to "incubate" and harvest dreams for direct problem-solving. She teaches them, first of all, to remember two or three dreams a week. When they've mastered that, they're supposed to pick a night when they're not too tired to prepare a dream journal. In the journal, they record what their day was like. The entry can be as long or short as a patient wishes. Next, they choose the issue in their life they want to deal with. They think and write about it as deeply and honestly as they can, framing questions to themselves about possible causes, dilemmas, solutions, etc.

Now they're ready for the trigger, a one-line question that gets to the heart of their predicament. They write it down. "Why can't I make my husband understand that he is overindulging the children?" "How can I improve my romantic life?" "How do I get my boss to understand my proposal?" Whatever the question, they're instructed to think about it over and over as they fall asleep. If other thoughts intrude, they're told to keep repeating their original question.

The next morning, the patients record as much of their dreams as they can remember. If they don't remember a dream, they write down whatever first comes to mind. And they're told not to try to interpret a dream right away. Instead, they're supposed to wait a few hours. If they have no dream recall, they're to try to think why that might be. And keep trying.

There are books on dream interpretation you can read, and you can also enlarge your knowledge through therapy. But bear in mind that this is still a largely unexplored and therefore controversial area. For example, researchers at the Massachusetts Mental Health Center in Boston, Massachusetts, claim that the form dreams take is *not* activated psychologically, but physiologically. In other words, if your alarm clock rings while you're sleeping, you may dream about train whistles.

Whatever theory is correct, there is one fact all authorities agree on: Sleeping pills disrupt the normal balance of dreaming and nondreaming sleep. As a result, they can disturb healthy mental functioning. Whether you keep a journal or not, it's healthier to dream.

Tired? Listless? How about some raw broccoli?

If you're down on pep, maybe the reason could easily be a lack of magnesium and potassium. They are the most essential minerals in combatting fatigue and keeping up your energy.

Experts differ over exactly how much magnesium is needed for health, at different ages and under different conditions. But it is easy enough to assure yourself of a sufficient supply, without having to rush out to buy supplements.

Instead—says Dr. Mildred Seelig of Goldwater Memorial Hospital, New York University Medical Center, who is president of the American College of Nutrition—make sure you eat enough foods that contain it: lots of raw or steamed dark-green vegetables, including broccoli. As for potassium, a banana a day will do the job. But watch your intake of alcohol. Liquor increases the need for both minerals.

What can you do for the boy who's a late bloomer?

In most cases, be patient. Male puberty usually begins between the ages of ten and fifteen, but not everyone gets there at the same time.

Delayed puberty affects about 600,000 boys. Doctors define the usual cause as constitutional delay, which can be attributed to a number of factors—genetics (there are families of late bloomers), nutritional deficiencies, and, though rarely, psychological problems.

To a boy, it can often be distressful to remain baby-faced when his peers are bragging about shaving and showing other signs of sexual maturity, such as body hair and genital growth. But he'll probably grow into it by his late teens.

If a boy has been growing in height by about two and a half inches a year but has not reached puberty by the age of sixteen, constitutional delay is the likely reason—and medical advice should be sought. The problem could be a hormonal disorder. That's easily treatable by taking the male hormone testosterone.

Some doctors believe testosterone injections should be administered at an earlier age if a boy is extrasensitive to his lack of development, or showing psychological, social, and educational difficulties attributable to his lack of self-image. Such cases, however, are the exception. The great majority of boys just need time.

Don't working mothers have rights?

Yes they have, and lots of them, too, thanks to the Pregnancy Discrimination Act of 1978 and other amendments to Title VII of the Civil Rights Act of 1964. Through these and other court-won gains, working mothers, working mothers-to-be, and soon-to-be-working mothers are guaranteed the same rights as men, regardless of race and age.

The problem is that not all women know this, and some employers aren't as forthcoming as they might be. If you're a woman who's looking for work:

- ☐ You can't be refused a job if you're pregnant. Employment interviewers can't ask about your birth-control methods, child-care arrangements, or plans for having children unless they ask the same questions of the men they interview.
- ☐ Unless sex is an absolute requirement (modeling men's clothes, for example), there is no such thing as a "man's job."
- ☐ Interviewers may ask only if you are between sixteen and sixty-five years old.

If you're already working and pregnant:

- ☐ You can't be refused a promotion or training.
- ☐ If the company provides disability benefits, you must be granted a leave of absence when you have your baby. You must also be offered the same job or a job as good when you return to work. You will suffer no loss of seniority or benefits. But, in order to receive these, the company may require that you work for it for a specified length of time. Maternity leave does not have to include maternity dis-

ability, however, because companies are not required by law to carry all-inclusive employee insurance. If you suffer a maternity-related disability, it is possible that you will lose your maternity benefits, so check into this when you ask about company coverage.

☐ If the company provides benefits to the wives of male employees, it must give the same benefits to the husbands of its female employees.

☐ While a prospective employer may not ask your age, once you're working your employer can—to enter you in the company pension plan, for example.

☐ Your medical, life-insurance, and retirement benefits must be the same as for a man. So must your profit sharing, fringe benefits, bonus plans, leaves of absence, and vacations.

If you're thinking of retiring:

☐ You cannot be forced to retire at a different age than men or to pay higher insurance premiums than men. Often employers will try to force this, giving as their reason that women live longer than men. It makes no legal difference.

☐ Benefits cannot be restricted to heads of household or to principal wage earners.

If you think your employer is violating Title VII and will not correct the situation, you can get in touch with the nearest Equal Employment Opportunity Commission office. There are fifty of them nationwide. Check for the nearest one in your telephone book under "United States Government Offices," or write to EEOC Headquarters, 2401 E Street NW, Washington, DC 20506.

How do you explain a college rejection?

With patience and understanding. Tens of thousands of hopeful high-school seniors are rejected every year by colleges they had their hearts set on. For many youngsters, it's the first major disappointment of their lives. They feel hurt and humiliated.

How to cope? First, it may comfort rejected applicants to understand that they have plenty of company. For example, almost 12,000 students applied to the Brown University class of 1985, but fewer than 2,500 were accepted. Most schools get many more qualified applicants than they can admit.

It also helps to realize that a college may make a decision for a lot of reasons that have nothing to do with the worth of an applicant. Most schools acknowledge that many considerations go into their decisions besides grades and class standing. Children of alumni frequently get special treatment, and it's no news that outstanding athletes often have a good chance of acceptance even when their grades are poor. Applicants from particular ethnic groups or geographic areas may have an edge, because many colleges work hard to keep their student bodies diversified. Even the planned choice of a major may tip the balance in favor of one of two equally qualified candidates. Hard as it is to do, the idea is not to take the rejection personally.

Experts say college rejection often throws parents for a loop, too. "There is a tendency for parents to identify with their youngster's successes or failures," says Dr. Everett Dulit, a psychiatrist specializing in adolescence at Albert Einstein College of Medicine in New York City. "When they succeed, it's one way for them to live out their own unrealized ambitions." Parents of a child who's been rejected should hide their own disappointment if they feel any. They can help most by being supportive and comforting.

College-bound students can reduce the risk of rejection by being realistic about their chances for admission to a particular college. High-school guidance counselors are often sources of sound advice about the selection criteria of individual schools, and can help steer a youngster away from an all-but-certain disappointment.

Students should also apply to at least one "safe" school where they are almost sure to be accepted. Youngsters who end up at their last-choice schools by default are frequently able to shine in a place where the competition is less. Excellent grades there can make it possible to transfer to a first-choice institution, or assure admission to a fine graduate school.

Painful as it is, college rejection can also be a valuable lesson in life's inevitable disappointments. As Dr. Dulit observes, "It is a part of normal development to learn that one's life—sometimes legitimately, sometimes unfairly—can be affected by outside forces one can't control."

Do the elderly OD?

Yes, too often, too easily—though unintentionally and unnecessarily, according to specialists.

Surveys show that the average elderly patient takes three to four drugs for various ailments. One study even found 14 percent of elderly patients taking seven or more drugs at the same time. One case exists of a person taking up to twenty-two prescribed drugs, plus some purchased over the counter, such as aspirin, vitamin supplements, and the like. Overdosing, or mixed dosing, is risky, sometimes fatal.

The nub is that older people often have more than one health problem. About 80 percent of them have one chronic illness, and half of them have two or more concurrent conditions. People over age sixty-five represent 10 percent of the American population, but they receive more than 25 percent of all medications.

The major health hazard is that drugs can interact, working to fight a couple of ailments but combining in a new and unwanted effect that can be dangerous. While this applies to everyone, the problem becomes acute for the elderly. Studies show that the medications they use are often absorbed and distributed in the body differently than in younger patients. Older people don't absorb drugs as effectively; their livers and kidneys are less efficient in metabolizing or excreting chemical products. Also, some foods will react to certain drugs no matter what a person's age is (see Appendix B).

So sometimes drugs can cause as well as cure sickness. In general, specialists say, adverse reactions to drugs appear to be more common in women than in men. And sensitivity to some tranquilizers increases with age.

If you're sixty-five or older, it's an especially good idea to keep a medication card, updating it with each prescription. Take it to your doctor or clinic on each visit, or take samples of each prescription, particularly if you are consulting a new doctor or new clinic. Talk to the doctor about any complications or side effects you are experiencing. Don't keep renewing prescriptions just because you can. Find out if you should do so.

Also, don't play catch-up; if you've missed taking a pill at the stated time, don't double the next dose. Throw away old medicines. Don't doctor yourself if you have symptoms months or years later similar to the ones a particular drug was prescribed for.

When to take a drug is very important, too. The American Medical Association's Division of Drugs recommends that drugs be taken at mealtimes or at other regularly scheduled periods. Poor memory and eyesight can be compensated for by having instructions copied in large print. The week's supply of a drug can be put in individual little containers clearly labeled as to purpose and time of day. Insulin injections can be premeasured and stored in disposable syringes. Finally, don't burden an elderly person with those difficult-to-open child-resistant bottles, or foil-packed and plastic-bubble drug wrappings.

Don't older people have rights, too?

You bet they do—more than many of them realize.

For example, a lot of people don't know that employment discrimination on the basis of age has been against the law since the 1964 Civil Rights Act, with additional safeguards provided by the 1967 Age Discrimination in Employment Act, amended in 1978. The latter protects workers between forty and seventy from arbitrary age discrimination in hiring, discharge, pay, promotions, fringe benefits, and other aspects of employment. It covers private employers with twenty or more workers, plus federal, state, and local governments, many employment agencies, and most labor organizations with twenty-five or more members.

If you think you lost out on a job, promotion, or raise within the last two years because of your age, you can do something about it. Get in touch with the nearest office of the Equal Employment Opportunity Commission, which is responsible for enforcing the law. Look in your telephone directory under "United States Government Offices." If there's no office near you, you can file your complaint with a U.S. Department of Labor Wage and Hour office, which will forward it to the EEOC. (By the way, it's illegal for your employer to retaliate against you if you file a complaint or participate in an EEOC investigation.)

Obtaining credit is another area where older people suffer from discrimination. It's against the law to deny loans or credit cards solely for reasons of age. Being retired or unemployed does not constitute sufficient reason for denying people credit either;

potential creditors must include any regular income you receive when they are calculating whether you are creditworthy. This includes Social Security, pensions, veterans' benefits, annuities, and public-assistance payments.

If you're denied credit, you must be notified in writing within thirty days after you apply, and the creditor must state the specific reason for denial—for example, lack of collateral.

You can also try to get a credit turndown reversed. A credit bureau or bank must tell you what was in its report at no charge if you request the information within thirty days of being denied credit. Because credit reports are not always accurate, you may be able to correct it or explain it to the creditor's satisfaction.

The letter denying you credit must also contain the name and address of an appropriate government agency where you can complain if you think you've been treated unfairly. If you're confused about which agency is the right one, get in touch with the Federal Trade Commission.

Age discrimination in employment and in getting credit are but two of the areas covered in a booklet, "Your Rights Over Age 50," available for $1 from the Circulation Department, American Bar Association, 1155 E. 60th Street, Chicago, IL 60637.

Does Linus have the right idea?

You bet. Having a security blanket, or a pet toy or doll, is perfectly normal—and in the long run, a child's early dependence on one, if the experts are right, may mean that later dependencies on cigarettes, alcohol, or drugs won't develop.

Research conducted at New York Hospital–Cornell University Medical College found that about half of the children studied had developed attachments for some object and that of these, half retained the attachment until at least the age of nine. The researchers discovered no differences in behavior between children who had formed attachments and those who had not, no matter what a child's sex was, how many brothers and sisters he or she had, and what the parent's marital status was. In short, the children who clung to security blankets were no less secure than other children.

In fact, the children with security blankets felt more comfortable in strange situations. They also tended to know exactly what they were doing. At first, the security blanket probably acts as an unconscious substitute for a child's mother. Over the years, however, the child becomes aware that the blanket helped to cope through occasional tough times.

Many parents express concern over continuing attachment to a security blanket and try to get their child to give it up. Often this has the effect of making the child cling still harder to the blanket by focusing attention on it.

Doctors report that a child will normally give up the blanket without prodding from parents when the time comes. Which means let the child decide when to throw it off.

When does natural mean artificial?

Often in the foods we eat. In some cases, the definitions of the words on a label are precise; in others, the words can mean whatever the manufacturer wants.

One of the most popular—and most confusing—words in use is "natural." There is no federal regulation governing it. According to the U.S. Department of Agriculture, many foods advertised as "natural" contain additives, preservatives, artificial coloring, or other artificial ingredients. The most commonly accepted definition of "natural" is that the food is minimally processed with no chemicals added, but deceptions abound. For example, manufacturers frequently advertise a product as featuring, say, "natural cheddar cheese." The cheese part may, indeed, be natural, but the other ingredients can include additives and preservatives. The only way you can be sure to eat foods that are "natural" is to buy fresh fruits, vegetables, meats, dairy products, and fish exclusively.

It's a matter of buyer beware regarding other food features, too. For example, the phrase "reduced calories" means that the product contains at least one third less calories than similar foods that a person can buy. If the label says "low calorie," the food cannot have more than forty calories per serving.

A "sugar-free" food, although it has no sugar, can contain an artificial sweetener that contains calories. If the "sugarless" food is not low or reduced in calories, the label must state this. A product may feature "no preservatives" but might contain other additives such as flavoring or coloring.

Finding how much sugar there is in a product can be tricky. This is especially true of sugar-coated breakfast cereals. The label does list sugar as an ingredient, but other ingredients might include sweeteners such as corn syrup, fructose, dextrose, or honey. Actually, the product may contain more sweeteners than anything else.

The words "fortified" and "enriched" also hold traps in understanding. White bread, for example, is enriched: Of the twenty-two nutrients processed out, eight are put back in. Although the product may be "fortified" with 100 percent of the Recommended Dietary or Daily Allowance (RDA) of various vitamins and minerals, the original product—especially if it's a grain product—might have contained more of these nutrients and a wider variety of other nutrients.

Although not widely available on grocery-store shelves, foods that are "organic" are usually those grown without synthetic pesticides, fertilizers, or chemicals.

A list of ingredients is mandatory on most food products, and the ingredients must be listed in order of weight content in the food. If water leads the list, it's the primary ingredient. So the best advice is to read all the labeling carefully, including not only the ingredients list but also the number of calories and vitamin and mineral content.

For further information, the U.S. Department of Agriculture offers a free brochure, "Meat and Poultry Products." It's available from the Consumer Information Center, Dept. 523K, Pueblo, CO 81009. In addition, *Eaters Digest,* by Michael Jacobson, is available for $4 from the Center for Science in the Public Interest, 1755 S Street NW, Washington, DC 20009.

The house empty without the kids? Want a suggestion?

Invite a charming couple from Rome for the weekend, make friends with a family in France, discuss Shakespeare with a Londoner, or brush up on your German with a businessman from Cologne. Then smile all the way to the bank.

Travelers in Europe have long saved money and enjoyed

homey comforts away from home by bed-and-breakfasting in private houses. Now the idea is catching on in the United States. If you have extra rooms now that the kids are off at college or on their own, you can meet people and make money by renting to travelers. The advantage of setting up in the bed-and-breakfast business as opposed to having a regular boarder is the variety of people you can enjoy entertaining, while having the option of doing it as frequently or infrequently as you like. What's a bargain for your guests is a boon for you. Some renters have made as much as $1,000 a month.

For information on how to get started, get in touch with Bed & Breakfast International, 151 Ardmore Road, Kensington, CA 94707. It now has branches throughout the United States, including Hawaii, and is run with a personal touch to ensure that travelers and hosts are carefully matched.

If you are interested in traveling yourself, but your wanderlust is bigger than your budget, you might want to find out about Traveler's Information Exchange, a nonprofit international travel cooperative whose members exchange lodging, paying one another a small fee to cover costs. Membership in the organization is $20 for the first year and annual dues thereafter are $10, for which you get lodging lists, a travel magazine, and the chance to meet with members. The organization also runs escorted tours abroad. Write it at 356 Boylston Street, Boston, MA 02116.

As for traveling in the United States, the Yellow Pages has begun a new heading, "Bed & Breakfast Accommodations," to list organizations that coordinate arrangements. The American Bed & Breakfast Association reports that there are more than 150 such organizations covering 1,000 cities. Individual bed-and-breakfast listings are expected to be offered in the Yellow Pages in the future. For further information, write the Association, P.O. Box 23486, Washington, DC 20024; (703) 379-4242.

Are you making sense when you talk to yourself?

Yes. And the most sensible thing you can do is listen. You've probably got something important to say. "I can't help but wonder how many good, creative ideas we throw out simply because we don't give them a fair hearing," says psychologist Shirley Sanders, clinical associate professor at the University of North Carolina at Chapel Hill.

Talking to yourself serves many beneficial purposes. It's a way of mulling over ideas, of making thoughts more concrete so they can be evaluated more objectively. "When we find ourselves verbalizing our thoughts," says Sanders, "it is a message that this is something which may be very important to us that we should examine and take more seriously." It's also a great tension reliever. For example, you can't tell off the boss in person; you'd be fired. But when you're by yourself you can shout away with impunity.

There are some instances, though, when talking to yourself is a sign of trouble—if, for example, it becomes frequent and the conversation indicates a feeling of being persecuted or being out of touch with reality. Or if it interferes with your life. Then professional help is needed. Another time talking to yourself is not healthy is when it results in a kind of negative self-hypnosis, when you keep on saying you can't do something so often that the prophecy becomes self-fulfilling. One helpful way to get over that, says Sanders, is to keep repeating, "I can do it. I can do it. I can do it." By which she means if you're going to talk to yourself, let it be constructive.

Can sunlight affect fertility?

Possibly yes, and in a most curious way. During darkness, the pineal gland located in the center of the brain secretes a hormone, melatonin, that seems to influence fertility, mood, and other body functions. In daytime, light traveling along the optic nerve into the brain triggers other brain centers to turn off production of the hormone.

It has long been known that light regulates the reproductive cycle and many daily and seasonal rhythms in animals, including bird migrations. Humans show seasonal rhythms, too, and these are more pronounced in people living at the higher latitudes than at the equator. Fertility apparently can be affected as well. For example, in Finland the conception rate goes up in June and July, when the sun shines for about twenty hours a day.

Humans produce more melatonin during long winter nights

than during short summer nights. Such long nights tend to depress people. Dr. Alfred J. Lewy, director of the Sleep and Mood Disorders Laboratory at the University of Oregon School of Medicine in Portland, tells a fascinating story of a man who suffered winter-long depressions that disappeared when spring arrived. Together with associates, Dr. Lewy, who then was at the National Institute of Mental Health, experimented by exposing the man to high-intensity light, mimicking the brightness of sunlight for six hours a day, three hours at dawn and three hours at dusk. In four days the man's depression went away. "In a sense, we made spring come earlier for him," says Dr. Lewy.

Recent research finds that humans are sensitive to the natural rhythms and changes in sunlight exposure from summer through the winter. So if you have to be indoors, open the curtains and let in as much sunlight as possible, and use full-spectrum light bulbs. But better yet, get outside. Ordinary daylight is still considered the healthiest kind of exposure. Take a walk on the sunny side of the street.

Is sickle cell anemia predictable?

Yes, and it's a good idea if you're pregnant and black to determine in advance what complications your child may face and try to avert or minimize them.

Scientists at the Medical College of Georgia have developed a safe and nearly 100 percent accurate test for detecting the presence of sickle cell disease in unborn babies. The test analyzes a minute amount of fluid removed painlessly from the amniotic sac, the watery vessel in the uterus in which the fetus grows.

Sickle cell anemia is an inherited disease most prevalent among black people. One out of every 500 black Americans has the disease and about 10 percent of the black population carry the trait. (It is also found, to a lesser extent, among people of Latin American, Mediterranean, and Asian ancestry, perhaps because the trait protects in some measure against malaria and therefore has been genetically conserved.)

The red blood cells of a person with the disease do not get enough oxygen and collapse into a distorted shape—sickle- or banana-like, instead of round. Because of their shape, these cells cannot pass easily through the small blood vessels and jam up and block the blood supply to various parts of the body. As a result, people with the disease can suffer a wide range of symptoms, including severe joint pain, jaundice, leg ulcers, impaired growth, heart or kidney failure, liver enlargement, and increased susceptibility to infection, although sickle cell anemia is not itself infectious.

The incidents of crisis are unpredictable and not everyone with the disease is badly impaired. Treatments through painkillers, blood transfusions, and surgery can alleviate the worst symptoms of an attack, and many people with the disease live relatively normal lives, holding jobs, having families. Research in recent years has provided new information and techniques for home and medical care that makes life a lot healthier and pleasanter for sickle cell sufferers.

What the new test analyzes is the genetic makeup of the fetal cells. To develop sickle cell disease, a child must inherit two sets of sickle cell genes, one from each parent. A person who inherits only one gene, from one parent, will not develop the disease but will carry the trait; it can, in turn, be passed on to the next generation. Two carriers, neither with disease, have a one-in-four chance of having a sickle cell child. Amniotic fluid studies are indicated only if both parents are carriers.

Further information about the illness and the test can be obtained from the Sickle Cell Disease Foundation of Greater New York, 209 West 125th Street, New York, NY 10027, (212) 865-1201; or from the National Sickle Cell Disease Program of the National Heart, Lung, and Blood Institute, Building 31, Room 4A-27, National Institutes of Health, Bethesda, MD 20014. Most large medical centers in urban areas or in areas with large black, Hispanic, or Mediterranean populations also have counselors on their staffs.

What's the reason for your baby's excessive irritability?

If you've been feeding your newborn a cow's milk or soy formula, it could be that. But don't despair: There's an alternative.

A recent study conducted by physicians at the University of Lund in Malmo, Sweden, concluded that both cow's milk formulas and, to a lesser extent, soy formulas may be a major cause of excessive irritability in babies.

In the study, sixty infants—all suffering convulsive abdominal pain, gas formation that distended the stomach, and the desire to suck often—were first given either a cow's milk formula or a soy formula. The symptoms of more than half of them either continued or worsened. But when the babies were instead fed a formula that contained hydrolyzed casein, all the symptoms disappeared.

Parents should keep in mind that colic, as such irritability is often called, is a common condition. It ordinarily lasts from four to twelve weeks, and doesn't seem to cause a baby permanent harm. Indeed, colicky babies generally grow and develop well. But if you are bottle-feeding and suspect your formula has been upsetting your baby's stomach for too long—and driving you bananas—consult your pediatrician. He or she may advise a change to a hydrolyzed-casein formula.

Do you really need another pair of shoes, that dress, those ties?

If the answer is yes, then enjoy your purchases and read no further. Likewise if you have an unlimited bank account. But if you already have forty pairs of shoes you don't wear and a bulging wardrobe complete with matching bills, you may be what psychologists call a binge shopper. Binge shoppers have a way of becoming debtoholics.

We all seek occasional pick-me-ups when we're blue or bored. For some people it's a drink or a chocolate sundae, for others the proverbial new hat or its equivalent. But binge shoppers, like binge eaters, are under a compulsion far beyond the once-in-a-while treat. Their debts mount and they become locked into a pattern of spending and borrowing, mortgaging future needs and dreams for momentary gratification. They know they shouldn't, but they say they can't stop.

The first step to breaking the pattern is to acknowledge that it exists and to recognize that it is not unique; others have it too. So prevalent is it in our consumer-oriented society that there is now an organization called Debtors Anonymous, which has worked out an effective program of self-help. The main steps in the program are like those in Alcoholics Anonymous or other such programs:

- [ ] Find a buddy, someone you know with the same problem, and discuss it openly and honestly. Work out a plan of mutual support to repress the urge when it strikes.
- [ ] Put those seductive credit cards away. Give them to someone you trust to hold for you. If you must, carry only one, no more.
- [ ] Keep a notebook always with you in which you record literally every penny you spend, just as a dieter records calories or carbohydrates. If at the end of a week you're aghast at the total, you're already on the way to getting better. Like eaters, spenders don't realize how the pennies, like calories, mount up.
- [ ] Make a plan of how you *really* want to spend your money. Think of your long-term goals—the children's education, a house, a vacation, a trip back home to see the folks.

Debtors Anonymous is a program of the National Council of Negro Women's Center for Education and Career Advancement at 198 Broadway, Suite 201, New York, NY 10038. Its membership is open to all, and there are branches in a number of cities nationwide. The organization will supply information and budget guides, or advise on how to start a Debtors Anonymous group in your community.

Also in New York City is BUC$, the Budget Credit Counseling Service, 44 East 23rd Street, New York, NY 10010, which offers free counseling services. Many mental-health centers and university and medical-school psychology departments throughout the country now provide short-term therapy for control of compulsive spending. They can help you buck up.

What should you do before moving to a new town?

If you have children, it's a wise idea to check out the schools.

It used to be that you could choose a good school district by its reputation. But with massive cutbacks in education, that's no longer true. If you want to assure your child of the best education available, visit the school district and satisfy yourself that your child's prospective school is all that you want it to be.

Certain criteria will help you make that decision. One is the school building. Is it safe, and does it have adequate space and facilities for recreation and extracurricular activities as well as roomy classrooms?

The number of children per teacher is important. A good ratio at both the primary and secondary level is one teacher for each fifteen or twenty students. The faculty should include specialists and a variety of supporting personnel and paraprofessionals to give teachers the time necessary for planning and preparation.

Elementary schools provide students with opportunities to read and to communicate clearly both verbally and in writing. They should teach elementary mathematics as well as fine arts, and offer physical activities and encourage the children's self-expression. If you're one of the many parents of young children who are concerned that the learning materials used in class be free of racial and sexual discrimination and stereotypes, ask to see textbooks and whatever educational guides are employed.

The ideal size for a secondary school, according to the National Education Association, is between 500 and 800 students—not too big, but big enough to offer a comprehensive and broad curriculum and an activities program. A variety of programs to meet students' intellectual, emotional, and social requirements is essential for a good secondary school. Junior high schools are supposed to teach children how to study; senior highs should allow students to choose and pursue their individual goals as well as encourage them to continue their studies through and even beyond high school. A senior high ought to have at least 1 guidance specialist for every 250 to 300 students to help achieve this.

There are other factors, too: the number of students in a class, the percentage of students who go on to college. For working parents with young children, after-school programs and public or school transportation are important considerations in making a choice.

If you want more information on choosing a school, the National Education Association will mail a free booklet, "What to Look for When Visiting Your Child's School." Send a stamped, self-addressed envelope to NEA Communications, 1201 16th Street NW, Washington, DC 20036.

Who says you go downhill when you retire?

Nowadays, hardly anyone. Not long ago, doctors and other authorities warned that retirement would bring on ill health, depression, and even early death. But luckily the experts have taken a new look at the data and decided that for most people retirement years can be pleasant and rewarding.

For example, Dr. Valery A. Portnoi, a specialist in geriatric medicine at Washington's George Washington University Medical Center, cites a study of 9,000 retirees that contradicts the common belief that retirement creates stress leading to early death. He also notes a study of 257 retired persons that showed that 37 percent underwent no change in health after retirement, while the health of a whopping 40 percent actually improved.

How did the idea that retirement leads to poor health get started? Portnoi thinks that some experts often fail to take into account the fact that many people who die shortly after retirement are in poor health when they retire—that, in fact, a large number retire because they are ill.

If an individual's health is good to begin with, it appears that most people can look forward to retirement without fear—an average of nineteen years of retirement for today's worker, an amazing quarter of a century for the one who retires in the year 2000.

All authorities now agree that there's one key to a happy retirement: preparation. You should start planning for retirement at least ten years in advance, perhaps even as early as age fifty. Here are some of their tips on what to do beforehand:

- ☐ Explore your local library. It's a mine of information about retirement planning.
- ☐ Take advantage of any retirement-planning services offered by your employer. Many companies sponsor courses and seminars on such topics as financial planning, medical care, where to live, even emotional and psychological preparation for retirement.
- ☐ Similar services may be available at a nearby university or community college. Take the time to inquire.
- ☐ Keep a file of all the things you've always told yourself

you'd do if you only had the time. These activities can form the core of your new life.

☐ Develop interests—sports, hobbies, community activities—that you can maintain after retirement.

☐ Force yourself to live on a retirement budget for a few weeks. Will you be able to cope financially? If not, start right away to get your economic house in order and guarantee your security after retirement.

☐ Make sure you and your spouse are on the same wavelength about retirement plans.

After you retire:

☐ Keep active. This is your best insurance against post-retirement deterioration, according to Erdman Palmore, medical sociologist at Duke University's Center for the Study of Aging and Human Development. "Those who retire to the rocking chair," he points out, "tend to find that their body atrophies for lack of exercise and they become withdrawn and often depressed."

☐ Keep up your social contacts, and initiate new ones. Work at friendships. Don't wait for others to call you; pick up the phone to chat or make a date to get together.

☐ Many people feel lost if their days have no structure. If that description fits you, set up new routines—times for work and for play, for solitary and for social activities.

☐ But don't get so busy you forget what retirement is supposed to be about. Indulge yourself. Sleep late if you've always wanted to. Finish the crossword puzzle for a change. Take your time, and don't feel guilty. You've earned it.

What's a woman over fifty to do for a job?

Your children have left home, you're looking for a job, maybe you've never worked before. What to do? Where can you go for the best help—and for free?

The public library is an invaluable resource, and an excellent place to begin. Here the older woman will find books on job-hunting strategies, some designed specifically for her, and also books on résumé writing and interviewing techniques. Some libraries have job-information banks as well, describing the sort of resources and employment available in the community. The library is the place to check out particular industries or sectors of the economy as employment prospects. It's also the place to find the names and addresses of companies that may be good bets for a job application, and the place to bone up on facts about an organization before going for an interview.

Midge Marvel, president of the small, volunteer National Coalition on Older Women's Issues based in Washington, D.C., offers the following tips:

- ☐ When writing a résumé, include skills acquired as a homemaker and volunteer worker. Describe them in terms the business world uses, such as family budget manager, church youth-group supervisor, March of Dimes fund-raiser.
- ☐ Don't list your age on the résumé; it's illegal for a prospective employer to ask for it. And play down the dates you held a particular job if it was long ago.
- ☐ Don't bring up your age in an interview, but don't be ashamed of it, either. Draw on the self-confidence your experience has given you. You've done things with your life, you've made important decisions, you're mature and responsible. Those are assets to an employer, and young applicants can't match them.
- ☐ Be well groomed for a job interview, but don't go overboard on makeup and obvious hair dye in an attempt to look younger—that can have the opposite effect.
- ☐ Take advantage of resources in your community. Many localities have agencies to help women and centers for displaced homemakers. Don't overlook the YWCA, which usually offers older women courses and counseling with career planning and job hunting. But watch out for the occasional shoddy organization that exploits the anxieties of people seeking employment without really giving help. If an organization's fee seems high, check it out with former clients, and call your local Better Business Bureau.
- ☐ Spread the word that you're in the job market. Tell everybody you know, and everybody you meet. Carry a résumé everywhere you go.

When is a safe driver a hazard?

When he or she is not alert to the signals from a medicine bottle.

You don't have to be an alcoholic or high on cocaine or marijuana to be a menace on the highway. Many normally sober citizens have not been informed or fail to take heed that their otherwise legal and beneficial medicines can make them dangerous drivers.

One out of every four Americans takes some kind of drug every day—to wake up, go to sleep, lose weight, calm down, stop sneezing, fight allergy, lower blood pressure, or ease pain. The drugs are prescribed by doctors or bought over-the-counter. Many of them can impair coordination, reaction response, judgment, vision, hearing, and concentration, make you "drunk," or put you to sleep. The antihistamines in cold and allergy pills, for example, are famous doze-inducers, while sleeping pills can slow you down long after you've wakened.

The National Traffic Safety Administration has ascertained that prescription medicines are the most common drugs, excluding alcohol, implicated in automobile accidents. In a study the administration conducted of five hundred injury-causing accidents, one out of eight of the drivers had traces of a legal drug in his or her blood.

The danger burgeons when drugs are combined with alcohol—even "one little drink." In another study, in California, of ten thousand "routine" drunk-driving arrests, it was found—not surprisingly, in view of the incidence of drug taking—that one out of four of the drivers was on a legal drug—273 different kinds of them.

Not surprisingly, the psychoactive drugs—tranquilizers, sedatives, anxiety reducers, and stimulants—are the number one troublemakers, often causing sleepiness. Also among this group are the drugs used to control epilepsy and Parkinson's disease. Valium users, for whom 30 million prescriptions were written in 1981, have a hard time following a straight line. They are statistically twice as likely to have an accident as nonusers, according to the National Institute of Mental Health.

Elavil and Triavil, two commonly prescribed antidepressants, reduce attentiveness and affect vision. Ordinary, mild painkillers called analgesics—whether touted for headaches, toothaches, or menstrual cramps, and especially when they are combined with codeine (such as Tylenol with Codeine, Empirin with Codeine, Phenaphen with Codeine, and Fiorinal with Codeine)—dull alertness and significantly lengthen reaction time. The strong painkillers—Darvon, Percodan, Demerol, and Talwin—are even worse in that regard.

Other drugs whose side effects can impair driving in some people include muscle relaxants such as Soma, Flexeril, and Robaxin; some ulcer medicines; high-blood-pressure drugs such as Lasix (if a patient's potassium level is too low), Inderal, Inderide, Catapres, and Aldomet, and some heart medicines. While many drugs are not in themselves depressant, they can potentiate the depressant effects of alcohol and other drugs.

Even when warned, patients sometimes ignore the warnings or take their medications incorrectly. Over-the-counter drugs frequently carry no warnings at all. There is a movement currently, spearheaded by the World Health Organization, to make such labeling mandatory, as it is now in some countries. So take heed: Avoid mixing your drink with a drug.

Does your body have its ups and downs?

If so, don't fret. Researchers have found that the body has a host of rhythms affecting its chemistry. These determine how you feel and how well you function. Called circadian rhythms (from Latin, meaning "about a day"), these "clocks" regulate such diverse body indicators as blood pressure, temperature, pulse, respiration, blood sugar, hormones, and heartbeat. Because body functions can vary as much as 80 percent depending on the time of day, an early-morning blood pressure reading, for example, can be deceptive on its own.

Doctors have found that the peak hour in a pregnant woman for the onset of labor is one o'clock in the morning. Heart attacks also come most frequently in the early morning. So do most road and factory accidents; night-shift workers in general tend to be slower and make more wrong decisions.

Similarly, a high-calorie meal eaten at breakfast can result in little or no weight gain, but the same meal eaten at dinnertime can lead to weight gain. This is because carbohydrates burn faster at the higher metabolic rates—or more intense activity—that occur in most people during the day rather than in the evening.

If circadian rhythms get disturbed by such factors as jet travel or changes in sleep or eating patterns, it can take several weeks before a new set of patterns emerges. This explains the phenomenon of jet lag.

Medically, doctors are studying circadian rhythms to ascertain susceptibility to disease and the impact of drugs. In cancer research, for example, doctors are looking into whether drug and radiation therapy is more effective if it's administered at certain specific times of day.

The key point is that if you are aware of the time of day you operate at peak efficiency, you can try to schedule your activities accordingly. Conversely, don't force yourself to face a difficult task when your body rhythms are at their low point.

Does jet lag have to be inevitable?

Not at all. At the very least, the disturbing shock of shifting time zones can be minimized; at most, it can be almost eliminated.

Most long-distance travelers suffer circadian dysrhythmia— jet lag—as their bodies try to make adjustments to radical changes in eating and sleeping schedules as the result of being plopped down in an environment thousands of miles away from and several hours different than their normal habitat. However, the effects can be minimized, medical and travel experts say, by the following guidelines:

- ☐ Begin your trip well rested and relaxed. Skip the bon voyage party unless it's held well in advance of departure.
- ☐ If possible, reset your body clock gradually before your trip. If your destination is five hours ahead of your home base, for example, start going to bed and getting up an hour earlier beginning five days before your departure, thus shifting back an hour to a new time zone each day. By the day you leave, you'll be on your destination's time.
- ☐ Starting three days before departure, alternate a day of greater food intake with a day of moderate fasting. During

the former, eat a protein-rich breakfast and lunch, and a dinner high in carbohydrates.

- [ ] Once aboard your flight, limit your imbibing to a single glass of wine with the meal. It can help you relax or sleep on a night flight. Also, eat moderately.

- [ ] Skip caffeine-containing beverages—coffee, tea, cola. They will make you feel more tired and depressed, and may slow down the resetting of your body clock.

- [ ] Get some exercise. Walk around the plane. Do some of the sitting exercises developed for long-distance travelers by Scandinavian Airlines: (1)"Jog" in your seat for three minutes. Raise your heels alternately as high as possible, at the same time raising your arms in bent position and rocking rhythmically forward and back, as you do when walking. (2) Improve blood circulation to your legs. Sit with elbows on knees, bending forward with your whole weight pressed down on your knees. Lift up on your toes, pushing your heels as high as possible. Then lift up on your heels, pushing your toes up. Repeat thirty times. (3) Rotate your shoulders and do head rolls.

- [ ] Allow time to rest when you get to your destination—a good night's sleep before sightseeing or business, or if possible a whole day before setting out, two days if you've crossed seven to ten time zones. If you've traveled far enough to reverse the day-night cycle, three days of rest are recommended, particularly if you're in late middle age or afflicted with insomnia.

People with some medical conditions should not fly at all, most doctors agree. These include people with collapsed lungs, severe emphysema, and serious heart conditions. Also, the American Medical Association adds, people with contagious diseases (including severe colds and flu), those with large unsupported hernias, and women beyond the eighth month of pregnancy should avoid flying.

Flying should be postponed in the case of newborn infants and anyone who has just undergone intestinal surgery. A wait of two weeks is suggested for both. Heart-attack victims should wait three to six weeks. In general, if you've been sick or had surgery, check with your doctor before checking in at the gate.

Because air pressure decreases as the plane climbs higher

into the sky, people with colds, allergies, and sinus infections often find that flying leads to sharp head pains. If you're suffering from one, try pinching your nose tightly closed and blowing it. That should help equalize the pressure in the nasal and ear passages. Decongestants swallowed shortly before takeoff can help, too.

What color dispels a black mood?

Would you believe pink? And not just any shade. Not scarlet pink or hot pink or pastel pink. But bubble-gum pink.

The color, according to many experts, seems endowed with almost magical properties. In San Bernardino County in California, the Probation Department places violent juvenile offenders in eight-by-four-foot cells painted bubble-gum pink. Within ten minutes they stop yelling and banging and often fall asleep. "We used to have to literally sit on them," says clinical psychologist Paul Boccumini, director of clinical services for the department. "Now we put them in the pink room. It works."

Psychiatric patients are apparently soothed by the pink color also. Today an estimated 1,500 hospitals and correctional institutions have at least one room painted "passive pink."

Another unusual effect is that the color appears to deter some would-be graffiti artists. In an experiment at Texas Wesleyan College in Fort Worth, children were put in pens of different colors. They scribbled and scrawled on the walls of all except the one painted pink. Cities, grappling with garish graffiti displays and burdened by lack of money to remove them, have taken note and are experimenting with the pink color in public facilities.

Chromotherapy or color therapy was once the province of Victorian quacks who roamed the countryside claiming they could cure everything from constipation to meningitis through the use of colors. Today chromotherapy has acquired some respectability as a developing science, though there are still those who are skeptical of what some researchers call "such a simple solution to very complex problems."

Colors are known to affect blood pressure, pulse and respiration rates, brain activity, the body's biorhythms, and behavior.

For example, when one hospital changed its walls from drab chocolate brown and gray green to pumpkin orange, strawberry pink, emerald green, and lavender, staff morale suddenly improved, elderly male patients started shaving, dressing, and getting out of bed, and female patients began asking for lipstick, powder, combs, and stockings. In another example, researchers painted heavy boxes white and light boxes black. Workmen moving the crates reported having more trouble lifting the light black cases than the heavy white ones.

How colors exert their effects is still a moot point. Do they simply set a mood? Or do they have a direct physiological effect, perhaps by stimulating the eye, sending impulses to the pituitary, pineal, and hypothalamus glands, which release hormones that control basic body functions and emotional response?

Color scientists say they have discovered some basic principles of colors other than those of the famed pink. Among them:

☐ Red excites. In red rooms, people's blood pressure, respiration rate, heartbeat, and brain activity go up. Muscle activity increases, as does the number of eye blinks. Restaurants use red to whet customers' appetites and to speed up table turnover.

☐ Yellow cheers and excites, though not as much as red. A local telephone company painted the interiors of phone booths yellow and found that people kept their conversations unusually short, freeing the booths for more callers.

☐ Blue soothes. In an experiment at the Elves Memorial Child Development Centre in Edmonton, Alberta, Canada, researchers repainted the walls of a schoolroom used by behaviorally disturbed children, from orange and white to blue. They also replaced an orange carpet with a gray one and changed the fluorescent lights to full-spectrum. The blood pressure of students dropped by nearly 17 percent and they became better behaved and more attentive. When the room was restored to its original condition, the children's blood pressure shot up and they became fidgety again. In London, Blackfriars Bridge, a favorite jumping-off point for suicides, was painted blue. The number of attempts declined.

Want to feel in the pink? Try it.

How should a do-it-yourselfer dress?

For the job—or you're likely to join the nearly quarter of a million Americans who end up in hospital emergency rooms each year, suffering from home-repair injuries.

If you're painting or using chemicals, wear goggles. If you're sanding or stirring up clouds of dust, wear a disposable paper mask. Wear rubber gloves if you're working with oven cleaners, corrosive or abrasive liquids, grout, or trees that have been chemically sprayed. Wear knee pads if doing any kind of floor work.

If you're working with power tools, don't wear sloppy or loose clothing that can get caught in the machinery. If you wear your hair long, tie it back.

Power saws in home workshops are the biggest accident culprits, says the National Electronic Injury Surveillance System of the Consumer Products Safety Commission. There were almost seventy-nine thousand such accidents in one recent year. A close second are manual tools—chiefly the hammer—which are also responsible for thousands of accidents sufficiently serious to require hospital emergency care.

Perhaps the most potentially lethal power tool is the lawn mower. You should make sure there are no rocks in your path—and no children or other bystanders around.

Almost twenty-one thousand accidents every year involve batteries, both automobile ones and the dry-cell types that power flashlights and children's toys. Most of the injuries are chemical burns, but a number are caused by battery explosions. Car batteries contain sulfuric acid, and the chemical reaction that produces electricity also produces explosive gases, which can be ignited either by a spark from the battery or by a cigarette. They can also explode when the do-it-yourselfer tries to jump-start a dead battery but gets the cables on the wrong poles—positive to negative.

Even the dry cells can explode or leak acid, causing skin and eye burns. It is wise to use protective gloves when working with wet- and dry-cell batteries, and hands should be washed thoroughly afterward. If acid does get into the eye, the eye should be flushed thoroughly and a doctor should be seen as soon as possible.

There are other hazards in do-it-yourself work. With improved insulation to cope with fuel costs, the home frequently becomes a source of indoor pollution. Cooking vapors and chemical vapors from cleaners are sometimes trapped inside a house. Use a kitchen exhaust fan and also air out your kitchen and rooms regularly. And if asbestos has been used to insulate the house, watch for flaking. Vacuum but do not try to remove or scrape off. Do-it-yourselfers should also take care in making electrical repairs. Homes built or remodeled between 1965 and 1973 often have aluminum wiring, whose connections loosen inside walls. Call an electrician rather than do it yourself.

Can a bubble bath be dangerous?

Definitely. And so can eye and face makeup, hair color, dyes, permanents and straighteners, nail polish and remover, shaving preparations, suntan lotions, beauty masks, face and body powders, skin creams, deodorants, and perfumes.

There are twenty-five thousand cosmetic formulations on the market today. Consumers snap them up to the tune of $10 billion a year. The Consumer Products Safety Commission estimates that each year they cause sixty thousand injuries to people's hair, skin, and eyes.

The Food and Drug Administration is charged with overseeing cosmetics. But unlike its authority with relation to drugs, the agency is not empowered to demand of manufacturers proof that the products are safe. Nor can the FDA require cosmetics makers to disclose their product formulas. Still, the agency and manufacturers say that most cosmetics are safe for most people when used properly.

Two products account for most of the injuries. Bubble baths can cause a host of problems minor and serious, including itching and skin rashes, urinary tract, bladder, kidney, and genital disorders, eye irritations, and respiratory problems. Children are particularly susceptible. Cosmetics experts' advice: Follow instructions on the product and don't use the sudsy powders and liquids to excess.

Eye makeup is the other big danger. Mascara, eye shadow, and eye liner contain preservatives to prolong their shelf life, but eventually these protective chemicals break down, making the products ripe for contamination by bacteria. Continued use of the cosmetics can irritate or cause permanent damage to the eye. To protect yourself, follow these rules:

- ☐ Replace your eye makeup every three to four months if you haven't finished using it up.
- ☐ Wash your hands before making up.
- ☐ Never use friends' eye makeup and avoid eye (and face) makeup testers at cosmetics counters. One recent study showed that more than half the demonstration supplies at a display counter were contaminated.
- ☐ Be especially careful to avoid scratching the cornea, which can cause serious damage.

Some general cosmetics safety tips:

- ☐ Keep containers tightly closed and store them in a cool place. Creams and lotions can be refrigerated to prolong their shelf life.
- ☐ Check the list of ingredients on packages to see if the product contains a substance to which you are allergic. With hair coloring and depilatories, do a patch test. Don't use cosmetics on irritated skin.
- ☐ Don't smoke while applying cosmetics. Some products, for example hair sprays, nail polish, and aerosol deodorants, contain alcohol, which is flammable.
- ☐ Don't mix half-used cosmetics or add water or saliva.
- ☐ Buy cosmetics in the small size. Date the containers and use only for the next twelve months, maximum.

Is overeating always the problem of the overweight?

Not always. A few people, because of hormonal or metabolic imbalances, may actually eat less food than other people but still can't lose unwanted extra pounds. But now there are blood and urine tests to identify and help with such problems.

One cause of hormonal imbalance can be the secretion of too much insulin by the body, which in turn may be an early sign of the onset of one type of adult diabetes. All persistently obese persons who are not overeating should be screened for diabetes, some specialists believe, because excess insulin promotes fat storage and may also cause feelings of hunger.

Other metabolic disorders associated with obesity include disorders of the thyroid gland and insufficiency of thyroid hormone; disorders and oversecretion of the adrenal gland, and—in adolescents who manifest poor growth and development, along with obesity—disorders in the production, by the pituitary gland, of hormones involving sexual maturation.

There are reliable blood and urine tests to identify each of these problems, and treatment is possible for all of them. But the percentage of obese people whose overweight is due to these abnormalities is very small.

The main usefulness of these tests, in fact, may be quite different. Many people who are overweight like to insist that they really eat like birds and that their trouble must be a "glandular problem." A careful physical exam and laboratory screening may identify the rare few for whom this is true—and force all the others, at last, to face up to their diets.

When is a vegetable diet just not enough?

During pregnancy. A strict vegetarian diet simply doesn't provide enough protein, vitamins, and minerals for a pregnant woman and her developing baby. She needs three hundred more calories than usual each day and an extra ounce or so of protein daily to maintain a healthy pregnancy.

Vegetarians who allow eggs and dairy products in their diet, the so-called lacto-ovo vegetarians, will have no difficulty in making the adjustment when pregnancy occurs. Nor will semi-vegetarians who allow fowl and seafood on the dinner table. But vegans, the strict vegetarians, will lack many essential nutrients. Even a carefully composed, compact diet of a wide variety of vegetables, nuts, seeds, legumes, and grains rarely provides the complete range of the eight essential protein elements, called amino acids, that are needed. Most such diets will not provide enough calcium and iron. None will provide enough vitamin B_{12}, needed to prevent anemia and spinal-cord damage in the fetus.

209

At no other time in life is so much at stake in terms of nutrition as in pregnancy. Additional protein is required to build the fetus's tissues and the mother-to-be's uterine, placental, and breast tissues. Protein is also critical for brain development and for producing blood plasma. Lack of it can lead to many problems, including mental retardation in the baby, toxemia, and even fetal death.

It's usually possible to get the full range of necessary amino acids from plants, but plant protein is not easily digested and pregnancy makes out-of-the-ordinary demands on a woman's body. So a diet has to be carefully planned. And while calcium—essential for the baby's bones, for the blood-clotting system, and the absorption of vitamin B_{12}—is found in soybeans, dates, apricots, and dark green leafy vegetables, it is difficult for the vegan to get enough. Supplements are advised. The same is true of iron, so essential in red blood cells.

The mother-to-be who is a vegetarian would be wise to drop some of her food restrictions in favor of a healthy approach to a special time in her life.

What should you pack for that trip to Timbuktu?

First of all, remember that you're going abroad from one of the healthiest nations in the world. The United States does not harbor many of the world's ills, with the result that you're probably not immune to many diseases found overseas—and you won't have a corner drugstore to run to in an emergency.

Take whatever medications you currently use, plus refills, depending on how long you intend to stay. If you are allergic to any medications, wear a wristband or a metal medallion that says what you can't take.

The American Medical Association recommends that you also carry a spare pair of glasses, if you wear them, and your eyeglass prescription. It advises taking sunscreen, cleansing tissue, sunglasses, foot powder, lip balm and water-purification tablets, too.

You should also carry a small first-aid kit with such items as adhesive tape, bandages and gauze pads, safety pins, tweezers, scissors, soap, insect repellent, and a thermometer. Common painkillers such as aspirin are also recommended. The AMA also suggests you jot down your doctor's name, address, and telephone number on a card, should someone else need to notify him or her.

Your doctor can provide you with some tips for your specific travel plans. A smallpox vaccination is no longer required because the disease is considered eradicated. Generally, vaccinations for yellow fever and cholera are no longer required either, although some African countries have requirements depending on whether your travels take you through areas where the diseases are active.

The best thing to pack is your common sense. Gastrointestinal ailments are common among Americans traveling abroad, largely because they ignore certain precautions. They can be avoided by drinking only purified, bottled water and by skipping raw shellfish or any fresh fruit or vegetable that can't be peeled. Otherwise stick to cooked vegetables. In case you do come down with diarrhea, there are medications that will relieve the symptoms. Ask your doctor which he or she recommends before you leave. And while the symptoms persist, drink plenty of liquids, especially fruit juices, and keep the diet soft, with such items as applesauce and rice.

The U.S. Department of Health and Human Services offers a booklet, "Health Information for the International Traveler." It is available by sending $5 to GPO, Washington, DC 20402. The International Association for Medical Assistance to Travelers, 736 Center Street, Lewiston, NY 14092, will provide free a list of English-speaking doctors on twenty-four-hour call abroad.

Are allergy shots the answer?

Some 6 million Americans apparently think so; each year they take repeated allergy-shot treatments. But a large number of allergists now think shots should be taken only by some of them—and only as a last resort. Conservative forms of therapy—the avoidance of substances (allergens) that cause an allergic reaction, oral medications such as antihistamines, or nasal sprays—should be tried first, they say, because some injections can cause serious side effects.

An allergy is an overreaction by the body's protective immune system to an otherwise harmless substance, called an allergen.

When allergens are injected in small but increasing amounts, the immune system is desensitized or made more tolerant to the allergens by producing specific antibodies to them. This blocks the release of histamine, the active agent causing many of the misery symptoms.

Before any treatment starts, allergists recommend a medical consultation that includes taking a careful history of a patient's living conditions and environment at home and work. Some have the patient keep a diary about substances he or she encounters and what reactions may occur. If the allergen still isn't identified, the doctor can give skin tests. This involves injecting tiny amounts of various suspected allergens through the skin. A person sensitive to a particular allergen reacts with a rash, redness, or hive at the site of the injection. The testing process, however, can be long and expensive before the right allergen is isolated.

The best defense against allergic woes, of course, is to avoid the cause, if you know it. People allergic to dogs or cats should avoid them. If you're allergic to down, sleep with a foam pillow. If you suspect some particular food, such as lobster, as the cause of a skin rash, drop it from your diet and see what happens. And if you suffer an allergic attack, try a medication before you resort to shots.

There are, of course, some cases when only shots can relieve much suffering, putting up a shield against the offending substance. Thousands of people allergic to bee and wasp stings—which sometimes cause quick and fatal reactions—are prime candidates for such shots, doctors agree.

Do nice guys ever finish first?

Yup, they do. For example, two hundred junior-high-school students surveyed by psychologists at Middle Tennessee State University in Murfreesboro were asked to rank several personality traits that help teenagers to get along socially. Surprisingly, so-called feminine traits—friendly, neat, gentle, nice—came out ahead of "masculine" ones—brave, tough, eager and adventurous. The researchers concluded that adolescents regard "feminine" traits as socially desirable—good news for the kind and gentle boy who wants to run for class president.

And if your teenage son would rather smile than fight, here's more good news. Such a youngster may be protecting his health in later life. Some traditionally masculine traits—such as being highly competitive, aggressive, impatient—are among those that make up what doctors call Type A behavior, personality characteristics of prime candidates for coronary disease. Thus, according to psychologists Dr. Nick Batlis and Dr. Arnold Small, "from the standpoint of potential physical consequences, strong identification with masculine traits without the moderating influence of feminine traits may be dysfunctional."

So nice guys, it appears, can have it both ways. They can finish first in the popularity game, and they can finish last in the game of life by outliving their hard-driving buddies.

When can marital bliss be all wet?

When it happens in the shower. For couples who enjoy sex, showering together is fun. And for those who experience sexual troubles, it can be an easy, nonthreatening, effective way to improve their communication and sexual relationship, according to Mildred Hope Witkin, associate director of the Human Sexuality Teaching Program at the New York Hospital–Cornell Medical Center.

Dr. Witkin advises a couple that has "performance anxiety" to take a shower together at least three times a week. Each partner is told to soap and wash the other, using hands, not washcloths or sponges, and to take turns toweling each other dry. During at least one of these sessions, they're advised to wash each other's hair as well. She encourages each partner to apply the after-bath powder or lotion, too.

One of the purposes of the intimate shower is to teach the couple that sexual activity is pleasurable without inducing anxiety about being able to perform "correctly." So Dr. Witkin advises the partners to avoid touching each other's genitals and breasts during the first week, and also to refrain from sex play and intercourse. Instead the emphasis is on relaxing and enjoying the experience.

During the second week, intercourse is still forbidden, but sex play can begin. A couple can progress to intercourse during the third week, although extremely anxious ones may need to postpone this stage for a little while longer.

Too embarrassing, you say? Most of Dr. Witkin's patients think so also at first. "By the end of the second shower they are beginning to enjoy themselves and to have fun together; by the end of the third shower everything has become quite pleasurable," she says.

So whether or not you're worried about your sex relations, invite your spouse into the shower. If there is a problem, you may be able to wash it away. If not, therapy offers a possible resolution of the problem.

What's the perfect exercise for everybody?

Swimming. It's the all-purpose exercise. It tones muscle, increases flexibility, conditions the heart and blood vessels, helps shed weight, and even relieves tension.

Swimming is so great for the body because it uses all the muscles of the arms, legs, and trunk without emphasizing any one area. And while it may seem to require no effort, it actually uses up calories at the rate of three hundred to one thousand an hour. You do work up a sweat, but the water washes it away.

Another reason swimming is called perfect is that it can be done by just about anybody. It doesn't matter how old you are or what physical shape you're in. Even those with chronic physical ailments can get in the swim. In fact, it is recommended for people with arthritis (it loosens stiff joints), backaches (it strengthens back and abdominal muscles), asthma (the air near the water is usually relatively dust-free), and varicose veins (the movements of the limbs through water massages leg veins and reduces swelling). Swimming can be especially wonderful for the overweight; their fat tissue makes them particularly buoyant and they can maneuver easily. And a recent study found that swimming is an excellent exercise for cardiac patients. Eight men, aged forty-nine to sixty-six, who had had a heart attack eight to seventeen months earlier were tested first on an exercise bicycle and then in a swimming pool. Fewer incidents of severe chest pain occurred when the patients were in the water. Oxygen uptake was also higher while the patients were swimming.

To derive any benefits, though, you must swim twenty to thirty minutes three times a week. Start off with five minutes of stretching or slow swimming to loosen up. Then swim vigorously using a steady, continuous stroke, preferably the crawl. Taper off by swimming slowly or stretching to end the session.

For safety's sake, never swim alone or when overtired or after eating a heavy meal or drinking alcohol. Don't plunge into cold water. And, when in a lake, river, or ocean, swim parallel to the shore.

If there's no water handy to plunge into and you're basically healthy—not suffering, for example, from back or foot problems, or a serious heart problem—another good exercise is jumping rope. It tones the body, strengthens the cardiovascular system, and aids in losing weight. But do stretch exercises beforehand, and wear running shoes and use a cushioned surface when jumping.

Who's a doctor's newest bedside helper?

A physician's assistant. It's a new medical career, an excellent opportunity for anyone interested in medical care.

Physician's assistants work under the supervision of doctors to provide preventive health care and counseling to patients, a particularly vital service in rural and underserved areas. They are trained to take medical histories, perform physical exams, provide emergency medical care, and in some cases perform minor surgery. PAs can even write prescriptions for some medications in some states. In fact, the U.S. Public Health Service estimates that a PA can assume up to 80 percent of a physician's workload.

The idea for PAs was born during the mid-1960s, when doctors were in short supply and some former military corpsmen wanted to convert their Vietnam training into a livelihood. The first PA training program was set up at Duke University. Today there are about 15,000 PAs nationwide, with some fifty centers graduating 1,500 new PAs each year.

A PA's education usually runs two years and consists of training in such basic medical sciences as anatomy and physiology, pharmacology, clinical diagnosis, and biochemistry. Training includes working with patients in such fields as internal medicine, surgery, pediatrics, obstetrics, psychiatry, and family practice.

PAs are certified by the National Commission on Certification of Physicians Assistants after passing an exam administered by the National Board of Medical Examiners. To maintain certification, PAs must take one hundred hours of continuing medical education every two years. Recertification is required every six years.

PAs earn about $22,000 a year, but this figure increases as the PA gains experience.

If you're looking for a career in medicine but the cost of medical school and the years it takes are prohibitive, write the Association of Physician Assistant Programs, 2341 Jefferson Davis Highway, Suite 700, Arlington, VA 22202.

Do you want your shorty to grow taller?

Sometimes it's just a matter of being patient—the child is a late bloomer. But sometimes, not frequently, it could be caused by either a thyroid deficiency or a lack of growth hormone. And now, thanks to a number of treatments, many of these problems can be helped.

Most girls grow to a height of five feet four inches, most boys to five feet six—and your pediatrician can tell fairly early if your child will reach at least that height. If you're concerned, the doctor will chart your child's height every three months to confirm that the child is growing at least one and a half inches a year; will look for signs of a serious or chronic illness that can stall growth; and, of course, will look at your family history. In eight out of ten cases, a short child will eventually grow and is just a late bloomer.

However, if there does seem to be a deficiency, there are now ways to pinpoint and correct many problems. Thyroid deficiency can be treated. And a new program guarantees growth hormone at a nominal charge to any child who needs it.

Many studies have shown that human growth-hormone treatment results in a normal rate of growth in children, and it's remarkably free of side effects. Until recently, however, only the well-to-do could afford it. Now treatment is available in about

216

ninety university programs across the nation for free, though there are charges for lab tests and some other services.

The ideal time to begin treatment is while a child is still growing—four to six years old—but even a sixteen-year-old can be helped.

So if you're in doubt about your child's height, if shoe size doesn't change, or the youngster's teeth come in late, have a pediatrician check your child's height every three months. If growth is below normal, a bone-age test can be done. This involves an X-ray of a hand and wrist, which, together with data about the child as well as hereditary factors involving the parents, undergo analysis. The result can indicate whether the child is growing normally.

If your child's growth is below normal, ask your pediatrician to refer you to a growth program. Or, for more information on the university programs, write the National Hormone and Pituitary Program, Suite 501-9, 210 West Fayette Street, Baltimore, MD 21201, or call (301) 837-2552.

What can you do to improve your child's reading and writing?

Make learning a part of life at home.

Many parents worry because their children are poor readers. Although television is frequently accused of being the culprit, educators believe that the problem is a family one, that it's not enough to expect a child to enjoy reading, for example, if you and your spouse don't encourage learning.

There are innumerable learning games and activities that parents can start to weave into everyday life when the youngster is old enough to talk. For example, say a word and ask your child to provide its opposite. (Start with "yes" and "no"—they're easily understood by a toddler.) Or ask the child to provide another word with the same sound. Have the child act out familiar stories, and encourage hobbies that promote reading, such as stamp collecting.

Paper and pencil should always be on hand and written communications should be a family habit. Teach your child to write his or her name, then go on from there to writing birthday cards, or notes about going to a neighbor's house, or letters to grandparents. Ask the child to write down the grocery list as you dictate it, or write the captions in the family photo album. Encourage the youngster to write stories or adventures; then pin them on a bulletin board and admire them. Children are immensely proud of their work.

Recent research has indicated that children's books need not have short words and simple sentences. It's more important that the subject matter be of interest to the youngster. Children won't learn to love reading if they're simply learning to recognize words that have no interest or meaning. The goal is to make children aware that what they read can be of use to them.

The next time you worry about your child's reading, take a look at what's going on at home. With a little effort and imagination, you may be able to turn your reluctant reader into a veritable bookworm.

Why are seat belts vital for mothers-to-be?

Because automobile accidents are the leading cause of death for pregnant women. Seat belts can lower the risk significantly. In a study at the University of Oklahoma Medical School of more than two hundred pregnant victims of severe accidents, the death rate of women thrown from a car was 33 percent. The fetal death rate was 47 percent.

Mothers-to-be sometimes assume that seat belts can be harmful to an unborn child. This is not so. A fetus, floating in the amniotic sac within the uterus—which itself is a strong muscular wall further encased in other layers of muscle and fat—is well protected from normal stress. The greatest danger in auto accidents comes from being thrown against the dashboard or windshield or out of the car. The impact of a collision on a car going fifteen miles an hour is equivalent to being struck by a two-hundred-pound sack of cement dropped from a first-story window. An unbelted rider cannot brace against such force.

Both the College of Obstetricians and Gynecologists and the U.S. Department of Transportation urge pregnant women to be sure their cars are equipped with properly fitting seat belts and to wear them. A standard belt is made big enough to fit around a four-hundred-pound man, so a pregnant woman shouldn't have any trouble with one.

Also, a pregnant woman who is in an accident, even a minor one, should see a doctor immediately and be carefully checked for several days after the accident. She should also make certain the doctor knows she is pregnant if X-rays are suggested; they can be a danger to the fetus, especially in the early months of pregnancy.

Even (especially) in the excitement of rushing to the hospital when the baby is due, put on that seat belt. It's a wise precaution.

How can you be sure the rhythm method works?

By adding new techniques to old ones to develop a greater awareness of when fertility can occur.

Many women—for reasons of health, convenience, or religion—would prefer not to use the pill or IUD, chemical contraceptive, or diaphragm. The only completely natural and safe birth-control method open to them is the rhythm system, which is based on abstaining from sexual intercourse during a woman's fertile period. As it has been conventionally practiced, it is not reliable. But thanks to recent research on the action of hormones, the regulators of the reproductive system, new approaches have been developed that, if conscientiously applied, can make the rhythm system more reliable.

Ovulation—the fertile period—usually occurs about fourteen days, plus or minus two, *before* the onset of menstruation, and lasts about two days. The old form of rhythm birth control depended on keeping track of ovulation days with a calendar, coordinated with daily monitoring of the basal body temperature (BBT), because in most women body temperature rises slightly (about .4° to .8° F) for about three days after ovulation. The problem is that changes in daily activity or sleep patterns or a slight infection can affect BBT.

What experts have now learned is that the cervical mucus also undergoes important changes at different times in the cycle and that by keeping track of those changes a woman can improve the accuracy of the rhythm method. As a result, some experts, such as Dr. John McCarthy, associate clinical professor of obstetrics and gynecology at the University of Pittsburgh School of Medicine, advocate a woman's learning how to test the cervical mucus as well as take her temperature.

Following menstruation, a new egg begins to ripen in the ovary as large amounts of the hormone estrogen are secreted. The estrogen also makes the mucus lining the cervix (the neck of the womb) very copious, slippery, and stretchy, to help the sperm along. The mucus is full of sugars and proteins to nourish the sperm. When the egg enters the fallopian tube leading from the ovary to the uterus, estrogen levels go down and progesterone levels rise. The progesterone causes the cervical mucus to thicken in order to prevent the entry of more sperm.

Women can learn to identify the quality of the cervical mucus, either manually or with the aid of new devices designed for this purpose. They can also test the sugar level of the mucus by using a special tape, called Tes-Tape, originally developed for diabetics. As ovulation approaches, the tape turns from yellow to blue.

Ovulation also causes symptoms in many women that are easy to identify: pelvic cramps, low backache, bloating, breast swelling and tenderness. A recent study has identified breast tenderness as the most accurate among these symptoms in pinpointing ovulation.

By combining calendar, thermometer, mucus testing, and awareness of one's own body changes, the rhythm system can be employed with greater assurance. Fertility-awareness kits are sold in drugstores or are available at family-planning centers such as Planned Parenthood. However, it's best to work with a family doctor or gynecologist to find out your very own rhythm.

Can peaches, cauliflower, and other foods prevent cancer?

There's a lot of exciting scientific evidence now that certain things we eat might help protect us against cancer, though it's too early to develop an assured anticancer daily menu. But the future looks good.

A big step toward understanding the possible connection between diet and cancer came recently as the result of a report by the National Research Council. It concluded that "it is highly likely that the United States will eventually have the option of adopting a diet that reduces the incidence of cancer by approximately one third." And the chairman of the NRC panels, Dr. Clifford Grobstein of the University of California at San Diego, says, "the evidence is increasingly impressive that what we eat does affect our chances of getting cancer, especially particular kinds of cancers. This is . . . good news because it means that by controlling what we eat, we may prevent such diet-sensitive cancers."

Backing the NRC study is a great deal of research over past years. For nearly a quarter of a century Dr. Lee Wattenberg and associates at the University of Minnesota have been seeking out anticancer ingredients in foods. He found that cruciferous vegetables—cabbage, broccoli, cauliflower, and Brussels sprouts—reduce the incidence of cancers of the lung and large intestine in animals given cancer-inducing chemicals.

At the State University of New York in Buffalo, Dr. Saxon Graham reports that people who eat cabbage as a main food have less cancer of the large bowel or intestine than people who don't. In England, Drs. Richard Peto and Richard Doll have found that foods rich in beta-carotenes, which the body converts to Vitamin A, are associated with lower risk of cancers of all kinds, especially lung cancer. Those foods include peaches, apricots, citrus fruits, the dark green and deep yellow vegetables (such as carrots), and the cruciferous vegetables. A twenty-year study of about two thousand men in Chicago found less lung cancer among men who regularly ate such foods than those who didn't.

In addition, Canadian researchers have found that, among more than a thousand women, the two thirds who ate beef, pork, and sweet desserts had about a 70 percent higher rate of breast problems than those who ate less meat and sweets. The breast cancer rate was higher among women who used butter at the table and fried foods with butter or vegetable oils, as opposed to those who didn't use butter at the table and fried with vegetable oils.

Japanese researchers have noted a rise in breast cancer among women of upper-income levels who can afford to eat meat every day, as against those who can't. Still another study has found the highest rates of cancer of the bowel in countries with the highest consumption of beef, and that includes the United States.

In an overall recommendation, Dr. Gio Gori of the National Cancer Institute advises prudence and common sense about what

221

you eat—try taking in less calories and less fats, in particular. The National Research Council has come up with the following interim dietary guidelines:

- ☐ Cut down the proportion of calories that you get from fats, preferably from the 40 percent in the typical diet to 30 percent. There is strong evidence that high fat intake is especially associated with higher risks of cancers of the colon, breast, and prostate.
- ☐ Each day eat some whole-grain cereals, fruits, and vegetables, particularly those high in vitamin C and beta-carotene.
- ☐ Cut down on intake of salt-cured, salt-pickled, and smoked foods like sausages, smoked fish, and ham, bacon, and hot dogs.
- ☐ Avoid too much alcohol, particularly if you smoke cigarettes. It boosts the risk of cancer of the upper gastrointestinal tract, and of the lungs and throat.

Something to remember is that while one in four Americans now develops a cancer during his or her lifetime, that means that three out of four don't. Something is protecting them, and part of that something could be in the foods they eat.

What's a grain of salt good for?

A cold in the head, especially for children. Many doctors recommend a mild salt solution for use as nose drops for youngsters with sniffles and runny noses.

Respiratory infections are usually caused by viruses, so antibiotics are useless against them. And common cold medications, such as commerical nose drops and cough syrups, contain ingredients like decongestants and antihistamines that many parents and doctors would prefer to avoid when possible.

Homemade nose drops, on the other hand, are effective, cheap, simple to make, and quite safe—*as long as you're careful to use the right amount of salt*. Stir only ¼ teaspoon salt into an 8-ounce glass of water. Boil the solution and pour it into a clean container that has been rinsed out with boiling water. Cover.

When the solution has cooled, use a dropper to put three to five drops in each nostril five times daily. If you don't have a dropper, dip a small piece of clean cloth or cotton into the solution and squeeze it to produce drops. Don't keep the solution longer than five days.

Speaking of salt, have you tried sugar to heal a boo-boo? See page 37.

What's funny about love?

That laughter will make your heart grow fonder. Laughing makes the heart beat faster, and that, experiments show, causes the opposite sex to appear more attractive. No kidding.

In one experiment, psychologists had men listen to a comedy routine. Those aroused by the humor, as measured by their heartbeat, had heightened reactions when they subsequently viewed a videotape of an attractive woman describing her life.

Other stimuli that make the heart beat faster work the same way. In another study, a film provoking anxiety—such as an Alfred Hitchcock thriller—made men and women more responsive to erotica than a neutral film that didn't produce physiological effects.

So if you're going to a movie, opt for a comedy—or at least a good mystery—and see what that does for your love life. Share your popcorn, too.

What's the peril in a peanut?

If you're allergic to the legume (a peanut is not a nut) even the smell can set off a reaction. And for children or elderly people with neurological problems, special care has to be taken about eating what doctors have labeled the Foreign Body That Most Frequently Goes Down the Wrong Way—down the windpipe into the lung instead of down the esophagus into the stomach. A peanut in the windpipe can cause respiratory distress, pneumonia, and other pulmonary complications.

For most of us, peanuts—by themselves or ground into a smooth or chunky butter—provide a tasty, inexpensive source of protein, and the peanut-butter-and-jelly sandwich is a staple of the diet of many youngsters. But peanuts are especially dangerous for small children, either because of accidental inhalation, or because they insert them into their noses, which can cause a serious infection. In fact, some doctors recommend that children under five years old not be fed nuts or seeds of any kind.

Peanut allergy is even more serious. Though rare, it can cause severe reactions—a generalized flush, hives, obstruction of the larynx, severe asthma, cramps, diarrhea, nausea, a sudden drop in blood pressure, and shock. There have been a few cases where people have become seriously ill because they inhaled near an open jar of peanut butter, ate a small amount of an hors d'oeuvre prepared with peanut oil, or shared a bottle of soda or kissed the lips of someone who'd been eating peanuts.

Children who seem to have an instinctive dislike of peanuts may be signaling their sensitivity to the legume and should not be forced, for example, to eat peanut-butter sandwiches. Because people with peanut allergy can also be allergic to other members of the same plant family, they should also avoid lentils, licorice, dried peas and beans, clover, and alfalfa. Children do not usually outgrow sensitivity to peanuts, although their tolerance may increase as they get older.

If you're severely allergic to peanuts, it's a good idea to carry an epinephrine injection—and for your doctor to show you how to use it. If you are exposed, vomiting is sometimes a relief. If not, get medical attention right away.

What old folk remedy relieves the itch of poison ivy?

Crushed plantain leaves. You crush the leaf and rub it on affected areas of the body. Several applications may be necessary before the itching stops.

The treatment was known as far back as the days of Shakespeare; in fact, Romeo advises his friend Benvolio to use the leaf for broken skin.

Recently, Dr. Serge Duckett of the Jefferson Medical College in Philadelphia conducted informal research using the narrow-leaf plantain. He found that the crushed plantain rapidly halted itching and prevented the spread of the dermatitis to other areas of the body. (The plantain did not cure the poison ivy, however).

Plantain can grow profusely in any back yard, and it's not as messy as calamine lotion. Your nursery dealer probably has some in stock.

When should couples discuss having children?

At the same time they should discuss finances, families, friends, and who does the dishes—*before* they get married. Not very romantic, perhaps, but very informative.

In an era purportedly marked by sexual frankness and openness in interpersonal relationships, it may be surprising to learn that many engaged couples have not talked together about the things that will most critically affect their future happiness: who'll handle the budget and determine expenditures; whether they both want children and, if so, how many; how parental responsibilities will be shared; whether they have the same interests, attitudes, and goals. And most are decidedly *un*frank about sexual feelings.

These findings reflect the results of a study of 38,000 couples in the Midwest and West conducted by psychologist Charles K. Burnett of the University of North Carolina. The couples responded to a 143-item questionnaire called the PreMarital Inventory, developed by Burnett in conjunction with a Catholic priest, an Episcopal priest, and a social worker, and based on their clinical and pastoral experience.

The PMI has been used with 200,000 couples since 1975. The responses are processed by computer and evaluated by clergymen or counselors, who administer the inventory and discuss the results with a couple.

Typical items on the inventory are: "My future husband/wife respects my wishes to pursue some of my own interests (hobbies, activities, etc.)"; "we agree that, if our finances are limited, television will be the most satisfying pastime for us"; "I think that my future husband/wife drinks too much"; "my future husband/wife is too dependent on his/her parents."

The results of the study shocked many of the participants.

Some of the women were startled to find that their potential husbands held chauvinistic attitudes about housework and child rearing. In general, both men and women expressed views of marriage much more traditional than might have been expected.

The overall response to the inventory was enthusiastic. Couples reported that the questionnaire opened the way to meaningful talks in which, with the help of the counselor, they were able to work through some touchy problems that might otherwise have caused serious problems. They were relieved to have these unsuspected disagreements brought into the open at a time when they still felt their options were open. A follow-up study showed that 10 percent of the couples questioned decided not to marry, as opposed to the usual estimate of about 5 percent in the general population.

For further information about the PreMarital Inventory, see your clergyman or a counselor.

Are strict vegetarian diets okay for children?

Usually not. Considerable research has documented many cases of malnutrition—especially vitamin B_{12} and zinc deficiency—and below-normal growth among children of strict vegetarians.

There are many kinds of vegetarians, ranging from people who do not eat red meat to those who eat no animal products at all. The stricter the regimen, the more likely nutritional problems are to arise. The strictest, diets based only on plant foods—vegan or macrobiotic diets—are limited in nutritional sources, and these can cause severe malnutrition in adults and children alike.

The vitamin most notably deficient in vegan diets is B_{12}. Research has shown that infants of strict vegetarians who were fed exclusively on breast milk showed symptoms of B_{12} malnutrition such as anemia, apathy, and neurologic abnormalities. Supplemental B_{12} can help these children, but other vitamin and mineral supplements are needed because the maternal diets are usually low in vitamin D, calcium, and iron, too. For bottle-fed infants, doctors recommend soy formula, plus supplemental vitamins and minerals, for parents who refuse to retreat to a less restrictive dietary stance vis-à-vis their infants.

In addition to nutritional problems, according to a report in the journal *Pediatrics*, the growth rate is "reportedly depressed" in preschoolers less than two years old who are on vegetarian diets.

Many vegetarian diets are close to the dietary guidelines put out by the U.S. Department of Agriculture—closer, in fact, than the typical meat diet of many Americans. But the strictest isn't. Avoid it. It can cause problems not only for your child but for you as well.

Guess who's got the postpartum blues?

Good old Dad, that's who. Depression is well known in new mothers, nearly nine out of ten of whom, a recent study shows, suffer a letdown, weepy condition and feel incapable and helpless a day or two after giving birth. But the same study shows that more than one out of ten fathers suffer from the same symptoms—though they don't recognize it as such but instead think they're suffering from a flu or virus or even dental problem.

The maternal version has been attributed to the fact that a woman's body has to undergo rather major hormonal changes in the six weeks following birth. She is adjusting at the same time to the responsibilities and demands of taking care of a new, little person.

But what of Dad's reaction? Some experts now realize that he, too, has to adjust, that the new responsibility in the house is his as well, that his role in the family seems to have changed almost overnight.

"It looks increasingly as if a number of things we assumed about mothers and motherhood are really typical of parenthood," says Dr. Martha Zaslow, a developmental psychologist at the National Institute of Child Health and Human Development.

The suggestions for solutions for both mother and father are the same. Talk about your feelings with others, including your spouse. Seek out parents of other young children for emotional support. Try to share the duties of taking care of a newborn so that neither of you gets so tired that you take it out on the other.

In almost every case, the blues fade away within a week. In the few cases where they are severe and linger, professional help should be sought as soon as possible.

By the way, it's estimated that 10 percent of expectant fathers—as many as 300,000 men a year—also go through a form of morning sickness and other pregnancy-associated symptoms. A man's abdominal discomfort, nausea, loss of appetite, and cravings for unusual foods are usually mild and short-lived, but nevertheless real. The cure? Identify the problem for what it is, a matter of empathy with the one he loves, and not the flu or some other infection requiring medication. Include the father in planning for the baby—shopping for baby things, discussions about budgets, childbirth classes. It's normal for him to have many of the same anxieties and concerns as the expectant mother, and he needs to express and share them.

What should you tipple when wintry winds chafe your skin?

Water, water, and still more water.

It is the water in your skin that keeps it smooth and soft. Some 60 to 70 percent of a person's weight is water. During an average day you lose about 5 percent of that water in urine and perspiration. In winter, water loss is exacerbated by the cold weather's winds, dry air, and low humidity, and indoors by central heating, which further dries the skin.

The best thing to do to keep skin soft is to replenish that lost water by drinking the liquid—at least eight 8-ounce glasses a day. Don't substitute sugared sodas, salty tomato-based juices, or milk for water; these liquids can actually increase your body's water needs.

Another bit of advice to keep in mind in winter: Don't over-wash your face and body. Bathing removes the natural oils in the skin that help retain moisture. Take shorter showers with warm, not hot, water. To replenish lost oils, drop some bath beads or crystals in the tub while soaking. When finished, pat, don't rub yourself dry. Dab on moisturizer and apply it everywhere—on face, hands, heels, elbows, knees, shoulders, throat. Be sure to use a moisturizer just before facing the cold outside. And a lip gloss as well.

If you ski, use a product that contains a sunscreen. The snow reflects 85 percent of the sun's ultraviolet rays onto the skin. Don't forget the often neglected spots: the nape of the neck, the nose, tips of the ears. Wear goggles. Male skiers should not shave for a day on the slopes because a beard retains the face oils that shaving removes, and also keeps cold and dryness from damaging the skin.

To help avoid drying out the skin indoors, lower the thermostat a few degrees. Use a humidifier or put some pans of water around the house.

To help remove dry, flaky skin, use skin clarifiers or exfoliating lotions. You don't have to use commercial products. Many of the ingredients in commercial skin lotions come from natural products—buttermilk, yogurt, papaya, tomato, lemon, and pineapple. You may prefer to soak in buttermilk, or wash your face in yogurt, or put freshly cut slices of tomato, papaya, or pineapple on your cheeks. If prone to allergies, however, you might be better off using the commercial products, which have purified ingredients.

Is it safe now to take estrogen during menopause?

Yes, if it is in combination with another female hormone, progesterone, doctors say.

Estrogen, touted as the "feminine forever" drug, was one of the most frequently prescribed drugs of the early 1970s. Millions of menopausal women received estrogen to restore their hormonal balance and relieve the distress that sometimes accompanies the change of life: hot flashes, night sweats, vaginal dryness, and pain during intercourse. The estrogen replacement therapy worked, but then a series of studies found that women taking the drug for prolonged periods—more than two years—had a four-to-eight times greater chance of developing cancer of the uterus than did women who never received the hormone. For many menopausal women it was a fearful discovery: Estrogen's risks suddenly appeared greater than any benefits.

Today, though, doctors say the risk of uterine cancer seems to be eliminated by giving progesterone along with the estrogen. In fact, the combination therapy appears to cut a woman's chances of developing cancer to half that of women who receive no hormone therapy at all.

The recent discovery is encouraging not only to women suffering menopausal distress. After menopause, many women develop osteoporosis, a condition in which the calcium in the bones is lost, making them thin and brittle and thus prone to break. Spinal fractures occur in 25 percent of women over sixty years old and hip fractures in 20 percent of women reaching ninety years. Estrogen is known to prevent calcium loss. A study of ninety-four women at the University of Copenhagen in Denmark showed that in those given the estrogen-progesterone combination after menopause for three years, the bone's mineral content increased by almost 4 percent. In women who did not receive the hormones, it decreased by nearly 6 percent.

Doctors stress, however, that hormonal replacement should not be used indiscriminately. They judge that only 10 to 15 percent of menopausal women really need the treatment. Many women can benefit from alternative therapies. For example, to relieve vaginal dryness doctors recommend the use of water-soluble lubricants during intercourse. For brittle bones, a diet high in protein and calcium and vigorous exercise can help maintain bone strength.

With all that's written about what to do about the problems of menopause, we sometime tend to forget that the vast majority of women pass through this period without a major problem and require no treatment and no medication. Fortunately, for those who do, there are now many more safe alternatives. So don't hesitate to discuss them with your gynecologist.

Is there a difference between play and leisure?

Very much so for a child. Nowadays play is often something that is initiated by a parent or teacher and resembles work. Leisure, on the other hand, is a time when there's really nothing to do and no obligations, and whatever a child then does is entirely his or her own idea.

Parents and teachers alike cram planned activities into school hours and afterward because they believe those activities contribute to a child's mental, emotional, and physical development. But a child needs leisure as well. As Drs. Douglas A. Kleiber and Lynn Barnett Morris of the Leisure Behavior Research Laboratory, University of Illinois, point out, leisure is more than just free time. It is freedom from the constraints of school and family, a freedom too few children have to pursue enjoyable activities on their own.

They urge parents and teachers to help children find leisure by not filling every hour with activities. They also advise parents to:

- [ ] Provide a stimulating environment. Make sure toys and other equipment are the kind that a child can use on his or her own, but help things along unobtrusively when necessary. For example, you can give your child paints in primary colors one day and then add more colors when interest wanes.
- [ ] Stay in the background. Encourage leisure activities but don't be the sole source of stimulation and inspiration. Resist the temptation to take charge. Boredom can actually generate play, exploration, and experimentation, but a child needs to know the process is under his or her control.
- [ ] Once you get an activity started, gradually phase yourself out of it. Leave control to the child. That will enhance the youngster's confidence, self-control, and self-reliance.
- [ ] Play *with* the child, which means treating the youngster as an equal—on the youngster's terms. Don't, for example, turn a casual session with a bat and ball into big-league batting practice.

A child needs time of his or her own. Providing it is one of the best and cheapest investments a parent can make.

What causes hives?

It could be a strep throat. Recent research indicates that many cases of hives are caused by infection rather than allergy.

In a study at the Geisinger Medical Center in Danville, Pennsylvania, almost 60 percent of the seventy-six children who had hives were found to be suffering or were believed to be suffering from a bacterial or viral infection.

In the past, doctors commonly believed that all hives were

caused by an allergic reaction to one of a number of possibilities—drugs, foods, contact with wool or soaps or other materials, even insect stings. Sometimes they are, and reexposure can bring on another attack. But frequently when hives are accompanied by the traditional signs of infection—fever, cough, sore throat, abdominal pain, or upper respiratory infection—the hives may be simply a symptom of infection and will in most cases respond to treatment with antibiotics or other medication.

If your child develops hives, and also pulls at an ear—usually a telltale sign of infection—or has a stuffy nose, a cough that lingers, or what seems like a weak bladder, consult your pediatrician for a complete physical, including a throat culture. If the cause is an infection, the youngster can avoid the lengthy dietary restrictions and drug treatment that people with allergies must live with. And a recurrence is unlikely.

Should you feel guilty about needing a painkiller during labor?

Definitely not, even if you're trying natural childbirth. Most women who are planning natural childbirth feel that if they end up taking an anesthetic or an analgesic such as Demerol, they've somehow failed. And they're left with a residue of guilt. But they haven't failed—and shouldn't feel guilty. If labor turns out to be unexpectedly long, difficult, and painful, they are actually protecting their baby's health and their own by taking a pain-relieving medication. In fact, not relieving the pain may be harmful.

Severe pain has two effects on a woman in labor. First, it slows the flow of oxygen-carrying blood to the uterus, thus reducing the fetus's oxygen supply. Second, it makes contractions erratic and unproductive instead of rhythmic and progressive. Labor lasts longer, and the fetus's oxygen supply is further reduced. The result can be a baby with poor color and muscle tone, one who has trouble breathing—ironically, the same characteristics seen in babies born to heavily medicated women.

Recent studies on baboons, rhesus monkeys, and sheep—all animals whose childbirth physiology is similar to ours—indicate that your baby may actually be born healthier if your pain and fear are reduced than if you grit your teeth and stick it out come what may. In the animal studies, researchers found that administering pain medication to animal mothers who were laboring under especially stressful conditions restored the blood flow to the womb and returned the contraction pattern to normal.

Doses of childbirth medications are lower than they were a generation ago, which often permits both mother and baby to stay alert during labor, points out Dr. Mieczyslaw Finster, professor of anesthesiology, obstetrics, and gynecology at Columbia University's College of Physicians and Surgeons. "With the epidural block, for example, which produces anesthesia from the waist down, the mother can fully participate in the delivery without feeling groggy—and she can feel secure that her child will be unaffected by the anesthetic," he says.

Only an obstetric anesthesiologist trained to administer epidural blocks can give them, and the woman who receives one must be monitored constantly, so the blocks can be used only when labor takes place in a hospital. Analgesics, like Demerol, can be given by the obstetrician. Small doses that will not affect the baby may be very beneficial.

So by all means prepare for natural childbirth—but also prepare for the possibility that you may end up wanting some medication. Discuss the types available with your obstetrician well in advance, so you'll have some idea of the options before labor begins. Practice your breathing and your exercises faithfully, and chances are good that you won't need medication. But if during labor you decide you want it after all, don't feel guilty. It could turn out to be better for your baby, as well as for you.

How young can a good Samaritan be?

Youngsters have had a bad press. The common wisdom is that they're all inconsiderate egocentrics. Not so. "Terrible twos" can be compassionate companions, and even one-year-olds are capable of altruism and empathy.

Guided by the theories of Freud and Piaget, many child development specialists have traditionally considered it futile to expect or encourage acts of sharing, kindness, or awareness of another's needs in children much under five, before the emergence of the so-called superego. But recent findings show that, to the contrary, kind children are not precocious exceptions. Dr. Marian Radke Yarrow, chief of the Laboratory of Developmental Psychology of the National Institute of Mental Health, claims that generous impulses are normal, even in very young toddlers, and can and should be cultivated.

Dr. Yarrow and psychologist Dr. Carolyn Zahn-Waxler set up a study of a representative group of twenty-four families. They trained the mothers in the group to record their babies' responses to displays of affection, pain, anger, sadness, fatigue, happiness, and kindness by people around them. Some of the babies were as young as ten months when the study began.

After nine months, some mothers reported that their children's behavior was a revelation to them. They cited one-year-olds eager to comfort (with hugs, pats, and blankets proffered); a thirteen-month-old who wanted to feed his tired father some of his own much-loved cereal; and another who tried to hit a throat swab out of the hand of a doctor who was applying it to his mother's throat because he perceived it as something that would hurt her. Kindly behavior extended to other children and little babies, and there was a great deal of sympathetic mimicry— an "ouch" when someone else bumped an elbow or brow. Although there were wide differences among the children tested, these were not related to sex or family size.

Psychologists and biologists may debate whether altruism is innate or developed, but studies clearly show that whether it's nature or nurture, it's there. Drs. Yarrow and Zahn-Waxler report that the most powerful influences on the children's behavior among their test group was the intensity of the parental message concerning the feelings of others and the degree of loving-kindness the mothers showed toward the children themselves—the hugs, the kisses, the tissues, the Band-Aids, the words of pride and encouragement.

In addition to encouraging positive behavior, it's important to explain why hurting others is unacceptable behavior. However, parents' expectations should be realistic. A normal child will often experience conflict between selfish desires and the eagerness to please.

Some parents may fear that fostering too much loving-kindness may not be the best training for a child who must make his or her way in a highly competitive society. But a large body of research contradicts the idea that cooperation and competition are mutually exclusive.

234

Are steam vaporizers effective?

No, according to recent research conducted at Tulane University. Steam vaporizers have no proven therapeutic value. And they cause hundreds of cases of injuries, mostly burns, every year.

The Tulane researchers noted three product-safety hazards of steam vaporizers: the possibility of burns from hot water, electrical shock, and exposure to bacteria, which may accumulate in the vaporizer if not properly cleaned. Moreover, inhalation of steam can produce severe pulmonary injury.

Many doctors now recommend the use of cool-mist vaporizers rather than steam vaporizers for treatment of a head cold or a cough. It should be cleaned daily. But no vaporizer should be used at all if the problem is in the lungs—for example, in the case of bronchitis. A vaporizer might make it worse.

A better way to fight a cough or a cold is to take hot lemonade, a lozenge, or, if a child is over a year old, a teaspoon of honey. All are as effective as drugstore preparations. If the cough or cold lingers, check with your doctor.

When are you likely to need vitamins?

When you're on a medication—prescription or over-the-counter. Some drugs, as a side effect, block the absorption of nutrients in our diets, so it's wise to know how what you're taking affects what you're eating.

For example, constant use of aspirin can rob the body of iron and may interfere with folic acid and vitamin C levels. Potassium and calcium are depleted by diuretics. Oral contraceptives containing estrogen can lower folate, and some reduce pyridoxine levels, which some experts say may be a factor in the depression that some women on the pill complain of. If you need to take cholestyramine for a lengthy period, chances are you're going to need vitamin D and folate supplements. And if you take mineral oil for constipation, it's likely you'll require vitamin D.

The problem is especially acute for elderly persons, most of whom are on some kind of medication. Many of them, for example, take aspirin for arthritis—and should eat a diet high in iron to compensate for the loss they suffer. And they'll probably need vitamin C and folic acid, too. Many elderly also take laxatives, which may decrease vitamin D absorption and, if the laxative contains mercury, may also deplete phosphorus from the bones. And that can aggravate the tendency older people have toward brittle bones.

What can you do? Simple. Make up for whatever your medication steals by taking a high-potency vitamin-mineral supplement or by adding certain foods to your diet. For example, for your iron needs eat liver, green leafy vegetables, dried apricots, prunes, whole grains, nuts, or oysters.

For other ideas, see the Drug-Nutrient-Food Chart (Appendix D) in the back of the book for a list of commonly used drugs and medications, what they affect, and how you can make up for it.

Is panic all in the head?

No. Almost 2 million Americans suffer from panic disorder, incapacitating anxiety attacks that strike out of the blue and that doctors for decades have believed to be a psychological ailment, an overreaction to stress or a forgotten past event. However, recent research indicates that panic disorder is not a disease of the mind, but rather a disease of the body, an inherited abnormality of brain chemistry. And two drugs now appear to be effective against the attacks for many victims.

We all experience fear when we're faced with a dangerous situation. That's natural and normal. But panic disorder comes with no warning and for no apparent reason. People with it suffer any of a wide range of symptoms, including breathlessness, palpitations, chest pain, choking sensations, dizziness, feelings of unreality, tingling of the hands or feet, hot and cold flashes, sweating, faintness, trembling, and strong fears—of dying, of going crazy, of doing something uncontrollable. Because the symptoms are so diverse, the condition has gone under many names: anxiety hysteria, anxiety neurosis, phobic anxiety state, hyperventilation syndrome, and atypical depression, among others.

Panic disorder almost always develops in the late teens or

early twenties and tends to run in families. About four out of five sufferers are women. And people with the disorder frequently develop other phobias as well. For example, a person who suffers a severe attack while driving a car may refuse to drive ever again.

Psychotherapy has often been useful in treating panic disorder. Minor tranquilizers, too—and, in complex cases, also antipsychotic drugs. Almost all victims have been given them at one time or another. Now studies at Massachusetts General Hospital and other institutions have shown that three other classes of drugs can provide relief in severe cases: the monoamine oxidase (MAO) inhibitors (particularly phenelzine) and the tricyclic antidepressants (imipramine and desipramine) and triazolo-benzodiazepine (alprazolam).

A recent study published in the *Archives of General Psychiatry* reported that patients often began to improve three weeks after beginning drug treatment. After twelve weeks of treatment, ten of the seventeen patients taking phenelzine were markedly improved and only one showed no improvement at all. Of eighteen patients taking imipramine, five showed marked improvement and all but two of the rest improved at least partly.

Dr. David V. Sheehan, the study's director, says the minimum effective dose of phenelzine is 45 mg a day, and imipramine's minimum dose is 150 mg. But both drugs are potent and the doses need careful adjustment, so he advises that they should be prescribed only by a psychiatrist experienced in drug therapy.

Reducing the panic attacks makes possible subsequent treatment of the associated phobias, especially by means of behavior therapy. So patients who begin drug treatment, Dr. Sheehan says, have every reason to hope that they may be able to lead normal lives again.

Are you fully covered?

By health insurance, that is. With today's ballooning medical costs, even minor health problems can rapidly strain a family budget. And not every medical plan provides full coverage.

Most Americans who work are covered by Blue Cross/Blue Shield, which will pay most hospital and some doctor bills. If you don't have such coverage—for example, if you're self-employed—the National Insurance Consumer Organization, a non-profit public-interest organization, advises:

- ☐ Join a Health Maintenance Organization (HMO). For an annual fee, usually payable in quarterly installments, you can see HMO doctors as often as you need to, get laboratory tests and X-rays, even be hospitalized. To find out if there's one near you, get in touch with the Group Health Association of America, 1717 Massachusetts Avenue NW, Washington, DC 20036, (202) 483-4012.
- ☐ Purchase Blue Cross/Blue Shield on your own. It is, however, expensive—up to $1,000 a year for an individual, up to $2,000 for a family.
- ☐ If you're young and don't mind large deductibles, try a comprehensive major-medical policy from an insurance company.
- ☐ If you belong to a professional or trade organization, ask if it provides low-cost insurance for its members. Many offer major medical, disability, and life insurance.
- ☐ If you can't afford any of the above, your income may be low enough to qualify you for Medicaid, government-sponsored health insurance for the poor. Check with your local social-service agency.
- ☐ As a general rule, avoid mail-order health insurance, cancer insurance, and nursing-home coverage. If health insurance is comparatively inexpensive, it probably provides poor coverage.

Medicare, the government-sponsored national health insurance for those sixty-five or older, provides a welcome cushion but does have some gaps. Medicare Part A pays for care in the hospital, in a skilled nursing facility, and at home. Part B helps pay for doctors and many other medical services and equipment, such as lab tests and wheelchairs. But Medicare excludes some expenses, including routine physical exams, private-duty nursing, custodial nursing-home care, drugs, dental care, eyeglasses, and hearing aids.

NICO says buying a Blue Cross/Blue Shield Medicare supplement ought to cover the gaps for most older people. If you feel you must have more coverage, insurance purchased through senior citizens' organizations such as the American Association of Retired Persons offers reasonably good value.

Medicare benefits change from year to year. For the most up-to-date information, the latest edition of "Your Medicare Hand-book" is available free at your local Social Security/Health Care Financing Administration office. Also available is "Guide to Health Insurance for People with Medicare," a pamphlet de-signed to help you choose supplementary coverage.

For consumer-oriented information about all kinds of insur-ance, including auto, homeowner's, and life, as well as health, write the National Insurance Consumer Organization, 344 Com-merce Street, Alexandria, VA 22314.

What do water and babies have in common?

They're made for each other, provided, of course, proper safety rules are followed. Like the womb, water can make babies feel safe and secure. And according to some researchers, it may even help them learn to make friends easily and adjust to new situa-tions.

Of course, we're not talking about teaching infants to swim. In fact, that can be dangerous. What we are talking about is learn-ing basic water skills, like paddling about in a pool and learning to feel comfortable and at home in the water. The emphasis should always be on enjoying the water, not on learning any spe-cific stroke.

However, it's important that parents receive instruction in just how to play with their infants in water. Accidents can happen much too easily. Your local Y can teach you what to do. You'll learn how to teach your baby to blow bubbles, to float, and how not to swallow water. Once you've learned how, you don't even need a pool. You can have water fun with your baby right in your own bathtub. Two cautionary notes: Be sure that the water is warm, and don't allow your child to drink too much water.

As the child grows older and wants to attempt more inde-pendent activity in the water, safety becomes even more critical. Drowning is the third most common cause of accidental death in children, and parents should be prepared to protect their chil-dren in water. Take a Red Cross water-safety course and learn mouth-to-mouth and cardiopulmonary resuscitation. And follow these water-safety guidelines: Make sure the tot uses water wings in very shallow water only—they're not effective in deep water. The pool should be fenced in and have lifesaving equipment such as poles and rings. And be sure it's you—not an eight-year-old brother or sister—who is supervising the toddler.

What's a help no matter what's the problem?

A self-help group. There are over a half million such groups in existence. They deal with anything, from drug abuse to divorce, from mental retardation to overweight.

A self-help group is basically a group of people suffering from like problems or difficulties who gather to give each other aid and emotional support. Such groups fall into three basic categories:

☐ Self-care groups for people who are suffering physical or mental illness or who are family to those suffering. Make Today Count, a group for cancer victims and their families, and the Epilepsy Foundation, for epileptics and their families, are just two examples of this kind of group.

☐ Reform groups for those with addictive behavior. Alcoholics Anonymous, Gamblers Anonymous, and Debtors Anonymous are three of the many.

☐ Advocacy groups for certain minorities, including gays, seniors, and the mentally ill. The Gray Panthers and the National Alliance for the Mentally Ill are two of the better known of this type. These groups lobby for legislation and social change but also sponsor mutual-support and self-care programs.

None of the groups are intended as replacements for doctors, psychiatrists, or other professionals. Rather, they represent extensions of professional care and sometimes adjuncts to professional care-givers. Some groups work with professional guidance.

Why the enormous proliferation of such groups in recent years? Alan Gartner and Frank Riessman, co-directors of the National Self-Help Clearinghouse, think the phenomenon is in no small part due to reactions against rigid bureaucracies and feelings of powerlessness. They say group members have experienced new energy, generated by being involved in a participatory process. And, indeed, joining a group can be encouraging, if for no other reason than seeing others with the same problems functioning successfully.

If you want to find a particular group responsive to your problem, you can often get names from your hospital, your doctor, or a health or social-service agency. You can also write to the National Institute of Mental Health, U.S. Department of Health and Human Services, 5600 Fishers Lane, Rockville, MD 20857, or the National Self-Help Clearinghouse, 33 West 42nd Street, Room 1206A, New York, NY 10036.

What's so good about brewer's yeast?

Just about everything. And if you're looking for a pepper-upper, it's much more nourishing than taking a vitamin supplement.

A byproduct of beer making, brewer's yeast is one of the best sources of B-complex vitamins. It contains sixteen amino acids, fourteen minerals, and seventeen vitamins. It is also 40 to 50 percent protein—one of the basic building blocks of the human body. Moreover, there are only twenty-eight calories per tablespoon.

The B-complex vitamins are active in providing the body with energy, but many Americans are deficient in this group of vitamins. One reason for this is that Americans eat so many processed foods from which the B vitamins have been removed. If a person is tired, irritable, nervous, or depressed, a B-vitamin deficiency may be the cause.

Brewer's yeast is available in powder, flake, and tablet form, but it is not all the same. Although brewer's yeast is the richest natural source of B-complex vitamins, it does not contain the vital B_{12} vitamin. In picking a brand of brewer's yeast, it's therefore important to make sure that this ingredient has been added. Check the label.

The easiest way to take brewer's yeast is in powdered form— one tablespoon of powder equals about sixteen tablets. Because a full dose can upset the stomach, it's best to start out with a small amount daily—one teaspoon—gradually increasing the amount to as much as four tablespoons a day.

One drawback to brewer's yeast is its taste—often compared with moldy dirt—which is why many brands are either flavored or processed to be tasteless. Moreover, when used in a recipe—for pancakes, or in a milkshake or orange juice—the natural taste of the yeast is overcome.

Is a warning label an aid or a hindrance in an emergency?

Better assume a hindrance.

Accidental poisoning is the fifth most common cause of death in the United States and the second most common childhood emergency. The most natural reaction when someone has inhaled or ingested a potentially poisonous substance, or spilled it on the skin or sprayed it in the eyes, is to take the time to read the label to see what antidote the manufacturer advises. Don't wait. Call for help—and act!

The New York City Poison Control Project examined the labels of 1,019 common household products. These included cleansers, polishes, pesticides, detergents and other laundry products, car-care products, over-the-counter medicines, drain openers, and plant and animal products. The project found that 85 percent of the label instructions were inadequate, incorrect, or downright hazardous. Twenty-six percent had no warnings and 31 percent did not list ingredients, making it impossible to determine what first-aid measures would be appropriate.

The most toxic substance found in household products, according to Dr. Daniel Spyker of the Blue Ridge Poison Center in Virginia, is methanol, which is an ingredient in some windshield-washer fluids, household cleaners, and spot removers. The labels on these products usually say to induce vomiting with salt water. But following that advice can kill you, Dr. Spyker warns. It's already happened in a number of reported cases.

Parents should instruct children, even young children, about poison dangers, whether solids, liquids, or sprays. And, of course, keep dangerous products out of a child's eager reach. Children account for 80 percent of all accidental poisonings.

When you suspect poisoning, immediately call your local poison control center (keep the number by the phone) or your physician. Give the victim milk, not water. Milk will dilute the poison without danger, whereas water can increase its absorption. Keep a supply of ipecac, a vomit inducer, on hand, but don't use it until advised.

As a result of the project's survey, the federal government is being urged to establish a clearinghouse to ensure proper labeling information. Many manufacturers are improving label instructions with the advice of the Food and Drug Administration. But at the present time you can't know in an emergency if you've got a corrected label. So call for help.

What will alleviate chronic diarrhea in an infant?

Eating. Forget that old advice that said a youngster with irritable colon syndrome should be kept on a diet of just clear (and often cold) liquids and low-fiber foods. That's not just old hat—it can actually worsen the condition by irritating the colon more. The best treatment, pediatricians now say, is three normal meals a day, and room-temperature beverages. But no snacks and no drinks between meals.

Irritable colon syndrome—sometimes called chronic non-specific diarrhea of infancy—is the most common cause of chronic diarrhea in children between the ages of eight months and three years who otherwise continue to gain weight and do well. Up to 70 percent of those affected are boys. The tendency may be inherited; relatives of affected children often have bowel troubles as well.

Most youngsters with irritable colon syndrome pass as many as three to six or more loose stools a day. Unfortunately, the condition does not respond to the usual dietary treatment effective in simple acute diarrhea; nor are over-the-counter diarrhea medications helpful. Yet one new study reported that more than four out of five children with irritable colon syndrome had normal stools within just a few days of being put on the regimen of three meals a day and no cold liquids.

Diarrhea in children can have many causes, so check with your pediatrician first before establishing the regimen. And you might as well know now: Your youngster won't like being deprived of between-meal snacks. But don't give in.

How can you expand your chest and grow taller at the same time?

By sitting down and standing up. If you do it right, it's a "mitzvah."

Canadian researchers have reported excellent results with an easy-to-learn, nonstrenuous procedure that they call the Mitzvah Exercise (from the Hebrew word meaning "a good deed that brings good to the doer"). In a study at the Faculty of Medicine of Dalhousie University in Halifax, twenty-five adults performed the exercise an hour in the morning and an hour in the afternoon. On the basis of a brief trial, their breathing capacity increased, chest girth expanded, and they looked, felt, and measured taller.

Poor posture—chin thrust forward, spine curved, shoulders rounded—causes a good deal of grief. Many Americans have chronic back and neck pains, often disabling sprains or strains. Many sufferers find it difficult to exercise, even though they know they should. The Mitzvah Exercise requires little physical effort, no supervision, and no fancy equipment, and you can do it for as long or short as you like, working up gradually.

The exercise was developed by M. Cohen-Nehemia, director for fifteen years of the Canadian Centre for the Alexander Technique in Toronto. He based it on elements of the Alexander method, which is widely used for reducing tension in spinal and other muscles, straightening spinal curvature, and lifting the rib cage. And he also has observed the Bedouins of the Sinai desert (who sit tall in the saddle). Here's how to do it:

1. Stand with back of legs close to a chair or, preferably, a stool, feet wide apart and toes pointed slightly outward.
2. Let head and neck fall and curl gently toward chest.
3. Let knees bend in a line over toes. Reach down toward the floor with hands between feet, sitting down at the same time and keeping the head and neck curled down all the while. Pause and count two seconds. (Less time at first if you feel dizzy.) Don't force your hands to touch the floor. Eventually they will.
4. Raise body to sit straight, chest and head facing straight ahead, hands hanging down at the sides. Breathe deeply for ten seconds. (Don't tuck in the chin.)

5. Let head, neck, chest, and back fall and curl down in line with the spine. Don't lean forward or backward. Pause five seconds.
6. Reach down toward the floor with hands between feet, keeping head and neck curled down, and pause for a second or two.
7. With knees in line over the feet, push the heels against the floor, keeping the weight on the back half of the foot. Raise body to stand up straight with chest and head lifted to look straight ahead, straightening the body, head, and knees all at the same time. Make sure the action is synchronized. Pause ten seconds. Walk around for a minute or two.

Feel good? You look good. Try it again. Just be sure to keep the head and neck curled down and the knees in line over the feet all the way down and up from the chair when practicing the exercise.

Who's Mommy's new helper?

The one in the diapers. Yes, it's true: Children as young as eighteen months are eager and able to help with simple household chores. What's more, they know they're participating in a necessary family function and they feel proud of their ability to do it.

What parents have observed at home has been tested and confirmed in a laboratory study at the University of North Carolina at Chapel Hill, where parents and children were observed and responses recorded and tallied. Psychologist Harriet L. Rheingold reports that children between eighteen and thirty months responded "with alacrity" to parental suggestions for participation in tasks and often initiated tasks themselves without help being solicited. They picked up papers, swept, stacked books and magazines, put away playing cards, and helped to make beds and set the table. Their ability to do the chores right was, not surprisingly, age-related. (For a two-year-old it's easier to pick up bits of dirt by hand than to manage a broom.) But even eighteen-month-olds knew, for example, that it's appropriate to put the cup on the saucer.

It's a good idea to start children in the habit of helping out at an age when they still feel eager to do it and get a sense of achievement in being part of a communal effort. Of course, verbal encouragement and the patience to accept a child's pace (and a less-than-perfect job) reinforce that eagerness to participate. It's difficult to resist taking over a task when you're tired or pressed for time, but if you resist the temptation, before long you'll have a very expert apprentice.

Updates

The following information represents the latest data and research into subjects that appeared in the first *FYI* book, published in 1982.

Wash and dry

We told you about the benefits of washing your hands to prevent your cold from spreading to others. Now comes word that washing hands is also a good way to substantially reduce diarrhea. A study at four day-care centers found that cases of diarrhea—the most common health problem at such places—were cut in half when the children and their adult supervisors washed up when they got to the center each day, before meals, and after using the toilet or changing a diaper.

Pain freezer

Ice, it turns out, is not only useful for soothing a toothache but also beneficial as a painkiller for, among other things, sore muscles, lumbago, and neuralgia. An ice pack wrapped on an arthritic knee, for example, relieves pain for patients who haven't been helped by heat or drugs. (And, amazingly, when the ice pack is applied for twenty-minute periods three times a day, *both* knees may become more flexible.)

Ice is also an appropriate way to treat a bruise. Apply cold compresses five or six times in twenty-four hours. This will constrict the blood vessels, keep the swelling down, and speed healing. After that, heat should be applied, also five or six times a day, until the bruise is gone. This increases the blood flow in the undamaged area near the bruise and removes all the blood that's gotten into the skin.

Ice therapy is a drug-free way to eliminate pain, but always wrap it in a towel, ice bag, or rubber glove. Incidentally, if you're up to it, soaking in a cold bath will often produce the same pain-killing effect.

A warmer choice

If you're not up to rubbing ice on your hand to relieve a toothache, try oil of cloves on the painful tooth. A panel of dental experts recently concluded that of the twelve active ingredients in traditional toothache remedies, only clove oil—or a similar oil containing about 85 percent eugenol, a clove derivative—was found to be safe and effective. Use it for temporary relief if the pain is persistent and throbbing, and be careful not to damage the soft tissue of the tongue or lips when you apply it. Occasional or intermittent pain indicates serious trouble. See your dentist about that.

Time and again

For those asthmatic youngsters who exercise but still need medication, there's a new drug that at least provides longer relief. It's called Theo-Dur and has to be taken only twice a day, at twelve-hour intervals. That's a big improvement over previous medications, which last no longer than six hours. Now the kids don't have to wake up in the middle of the night to take a dose, and are less likely, also, to forget about taking their medicine during the day.

And for those kids and adults who suffer exercise-induced asthma (EIA) when playing outdoors in the winter, there are now medications that can be inhaled, and an even simpler solution— a mouth-and-nose mask. According to Dr. E. Neil Schachter, director of respiratory therapy at Yale New Haven Medical Center, it doesn't matter if the mask is one of those especially made for cold weather or a common dust mask; either can moderate the air entering the body, enough, says Dr. Schachter, to weaken and in some cases completely prevent EIA. A mask is a good idea, too, for the many asthmatic joggers and cross-country skiers who find themselves wheezing and short of breath when the temperature and humidity drop and their breathing rate increases, cooling and drying their airways.

Attention, pill takers

Even if you watch what you drink when you take any pill, you can still be missing out on quick relief—unless you stand up. Army investigators have found that lying down tends to trap medication in the esophagus for five minutes or longer, delaying its reaching the stomach and being absorbed into the bloodstream. Many drugs—including antibiotics, iron tablets, quinidine, and vitamin C—can irritate the esophagus, causing burning pain and difficulty in swallowing. So always wash down a pill with liquid—water, juice, or whatever the doctor advises—and if you're not confined to bed, stand up for a couple of minutes to enable it to get down to work.

The point of it all

If you've found that acupressure works for your headaches, stomachaches, and the like, here's what to do if you suffer from sinusitis:

First, blow your nose gently, without pinching the nostrils. Then, in sequence, apply pressure to the following spots: the top of the head at the center of the skull in a direct line above the nose, at the hairline in a direct line above the nose, in the center of the forehead directly above the nose, on both sides of the nose at the point where it widens just below the bridge, on the upper gums at both sides of the nostrils, and both sides of the jawline at the point where it starts to widen toward the jawbone. Repeat the full cycle two to four times.

When applying pressure, don't forget to vibrate as you push down on the pressure point, then rotate your finger rapidly, always clockwise.

Want to see if acupressure can work for you? Put your index fingers tip to tip in front of you, about chest high. Ask a friend to pull them apart while you force the tips together; it shouldn't be possible. Now have your friend massage the sides of your forehead, behind each eye, gently for a few seconds. Ask the friend to try again to pull the fingers apart. No matter how hard you resist, the fingers should part easily.

There's another easy illustration. Extend an arm straight out. Have your friend try to force it down while you resist. That shouldn't work either, so have your friend gently massage behind the ear on the same side as the arm, then try to press down your arm. That should do it.

Picture this

There's a new suggestion to soothe a young child when you want to go out: Leave a photograph of Mom. Youngsters relax when they have a shot of Mom in hand, according to a study on separation distress by the Department of Psychology at the University of Wisconsin. The visual perception enables children as young as twenty months to overcome being upset.And don't forget, there's always that game of peek-a-boo, too.

Surgery bypass

Remember we told you how heart attacks can be prevented if warning signals—chest pain, pain in the left arm, dizziness, fainting—are heeded? That you should seek help immediately? That still holds. But if a heart attack is caused because a blood clot has blocked a coronary artery, a new procedure using the drug streptokinase may dissolve the clot and stop the attack.

In one study it prevented first-time attacks 90 percent of the time, and reduced by about 50 percent the number of patients requiring coronary bypass surgery. But remember to heed the warning signs of a heart attack—you still must get to a hospital quickly to benefit from streptokinase.

The drug has only recently been approved by the Food and Drug Administration. Although it is available at most major medical centers, it is still undergoing tests. Check with a doctor for the latest information.

Tum-tum treatment

There are now new drugs besides cimetidine (Tagamet) for treating ulcers. One is Zantac. A major factor in its favor is that it requires fewer daily doses than cimetidine does. Another new medication is sucralfate, which works by forming a protective coating over an ulcer. Still another, Ranitidine, is expected to win FDA approval by the end of 1983.

Also, Dr. William M. Steinberg of the George Washington University Medical Center cautions patients with peptic ulcers not to take a commercial antacid at the same time as cimetidine (which is usually taken at mealtimes); the latter's effectiveness declines. Instead, he advises that the antacid be taken an hour before the cimetidine. Of course, check with your doctor about these new alternatives.

Acne relief

A new medication is available from dermatologists, who up to now have advised the use of benzoyl peroxide, antibiotics, and sulfur to treat acne. It's Accutane, a synthetic chemical related to vitamin A, and is said to be nearly 100 percent effective in clearing up serious cases of acne. Almost all of the five hundred people it was tested on showed either marked improvement or complete recovery from the unsightly affliction. It is taken internally, in capsule form.

Accutane may have side effects and is not recommended for pregnant women because of possible risk to the fetus.

Living for two

The latest advice on the pregnancy-nutrition front is that mothers-to-be can and should indulge that fantasy of a lifetime, snacking whenever they feel like it, provided the snacks are healthy and nutritious. That's because a fetus eats around the clock.

Even if a woman who is pregnant is overweight, doctors now advise that she gain at least fifteen pounds. Breakfast is especially important. If a woman skips it, her body usually does not have enough sugar to use as energy, and other sources, fat and protein, are used instead. This results in an increase of ketones and lipids in the blood, which, if passed to the fetus, could be harmful. So start the day eating for two. And it's a good idea to have a bedtime snack, too.

As for those annoying leg cramps that many pregnant women complain about, calcium supplements may be the answer. Norwegian scientists have found that taking the supplements over a two-week period eased or eliminated the cramps entirely. They theorize that the cramps are caused by the gradual decrease in certain calcium complexes during pregnancy.

In addition, it appears that women in the last weeks of pregnancy would do better to take acetaminophen rather than aspirin when they have a headache. According to a study reported in the journal *Obstetrics and Gynecology,* there's a connection between the use of aspirin in late pregnancy and intracranial hemorrhage in infants.

And there's also evidence that women who do take aspirin late in their term face prolonged gestation and labor as well as excessive blood loss during delivery. In a study at the Upstate Medical Center in Syracuse, New York, unusual and excessive bleeding, mostly in the form of skin hemorrhages, was also found in babies whose mothers had taken aspirin within five days of giving birth. Worried because nearly seven out of ten women are known to take aspirin sometime during the last three months of pregnancy, the researchers urge that aspirin be avoided entirely *throughout* a pregnancy.

Similarly, some health authorities are now warning mothers-to-be against taking many of the thousands of over-the-counter medications available in drugstores and food stores. Antihistamines, they say, may harm the fetus or the nursing infant. They also caution pregnant women to stay away from alcohol; an ounce a day, they point out, *may* lead to a significant decrease in a baby's weight at birth, and as little as half an ounce can increase the likelihood of spontaneous abortion. Coffee should be taken in moderation (because of the caffeine).

One thing a pregnant woman can do for herself without resorting to drugs is get enough sleep, whether in the early or late part of the term. In the early months, the body's adjustment to the pregnancy often makes sleep difficult; in the last few months, a woman is frequently kept awake because of her increased size, increased bladder pressure, or the fetus's kicking. To get a good night's sleep:

☐ Take a warm bath before going to bed.
☐ Drink warm milk before bedtime.
☐ Do childbirth exercises or other relaxation techniques.
☐ Avoid caffeine in any form—coffee, soft drinks, etc.

A guide to a drug-free pregnancy, "Safe Natural Remedies for Discomforts of Pregnancy," can be obtained for $1.50 plus 50 cents postage from the OTC (Over-the-Counter) Drug Committee, Coalition for the Medical Rights of Women, 1638-B Haight Street, San Francisco, CA 94117.

Double takes

If you've come up negative on one of those home pregnancy tests, try again. One study shows that a false finding occurs in nearly a fourth of all negative results.

Part of the problem, Dr. Barbara G. Valanis and Carol S. Perlman report in a recent issue of the *American Journal of Public Health,* is that almost two thirds of the women who use test kits fail to follow instructions: They either take the test before the recommended nine days or they don't bother to take a second one to confirm a negative result.

That could be bad news; a woman who doesn't think she's pregnant will probably continue drinking, smoking, and ignoring her diet—all detrimental to the fetus. Alcohol alone, a spokesman for the U.S. Department of Health and Human Services says, affects one in every six hundred babies, causing severe birth defects such as smaller-than-normal babies, very small head size, and mental retardation.

What is important, therefore, is to retest yourself one week later if you still haven't menstruated.

All the way

The importance of finishing all the medicine a doctor prescribes is critical for children who are taking an antibiotic for strep throat. It's essential that they continue on the antibiotic for at least ten days, no matter how much better they feel after a day or so. Otherwise, according to a new warning from the American Academy of Pediatrics, the strep infection could still be present, and complications—a middle-ear infection, rheumatic fever, kidney disease, or a heart infection called endocarditis—are possible.

Bedtime story

There's more evidence about the fallacy of relying on a sleeping pill every night. Even though we Americans take enough of them every year to put all 230 million of us to sleep for two hundred hours, the people who actually turn to a pill for help are not only sleeping less and taking more, they're very likely to be endangering their lives. These so-called hypnotic drugs can interfere with a person's natural arousal defense in the dark, the ability to wake up if something goes wrong. And sleeping pills have been implicated in a third of all drug-related deaths, whether they're intentional (suicide) or accidental. They're especially lethal in combination with liquor and for older adults, whose bodies ordinarily need more time to break down drugs.

For those who suffer deep-seated fatigue, edginess, headaches, muscle spasms, and nausea, there's a simple method of relaxation that takes less than fifteen minutes a day. It's called Progressive Relaxation and involves the tensing and relaxing of muscle groups all over the body. To do it, first find a quiet room away from distractions. It should have a bed, couch, or padded mat, but an easy chair or ottoman will do, too. Loosen any tight-fitting clothing and lie on your back, trying to be as totally relaxed as possible. Get as comfortable as possible; if lying on the floor, put pillows under your knees and neck. Now, with your eyes closed, breathe deeply, slowly exhaling, for a minute or so. Next, starting with your right foot, clench your toes and take a deep, slow breath, trying all the while to tighten all the muscles in your foot. Let the muscles go and exhale after ten to fifteen seconds, relaxing as you do so. Breathe easily for half a minute, then repeat. Follow the same procedure for the calves, thighs, buttocks, abdominal muscles, chest, upper back, hands, forearms, upper arms, neck, then jaw and facial muscles—in that order.

The Progressive Relaxation method should be practiced in bed before you go to sleep and at least once during the day if your tension level is high. After a while it should become like a conditioned reflex; your muscles become capable of sensing excess tension and triggering a relaxation response.

In a pinch

Leg cramps are not the only discomfort that acupinch will relieve, according to its discoverer, Milton F. Allen. He says the broad, sustained pinch of the upper lip area, between the nose and upper lip, has been cited by numerous sufferers in helping to relieve, among other nuisances, hiccups, muscle cramps during pregnancy, lower back spasms, cramps caused by varicose veins, and rectal cramps. Several persons say they've been able to eliminate cramps during swimming and driving by means of acupinch.

More medicinal advice

Aware that patients find it difficult to get accurate and total information about the drugs they take, the American Medical Association has started a major program to provide easy-to-read leaflets about the most widely used medicines. Called "Patient

Medication Instructions," the leaflets are being distributed free through doctors. The drugs covered will include tranquilizers, insulin, oral penicillin, and nitroglycerin. Information about sixty such drugs is now available, and that number should reach one hundred by 1984. If you get a prescription from a doctor, ask for a PMI to take with you, too.

The U.S. Pharmacopeial Convention, which is cooperating with the AMA effort, also publishes a bimonthly newsletter called "About Your Medicines." A subscription costs $3 from the convention's Drug Information Division, 12601 Twinbrook Parkway, Rockville, MD 20852.

Merchandise complaints

Add to the ways you can fight back against unwanted mail-order and store goods the fact that you do not have to return or pay for any goods received in the U.S. mail if you didn't order them. That goes, says the Federal Trade Commission, for merchandise sent "on approval" without your permission, the receipt of products different from what you ordered, and the failure of companies to stop sending merchandise if you cancel a purchase plan.

Almost-free for all

Add to the list of federal and municipal agencies that sponsor auctions the Internal Revenue Service. It sells items seized from individuals or businesses for nonpayment of taxes—and that can include cars, boats, furniture, other household goods, real estate. Often they go for half or less of wholesale value. Each IRS district office has a regional mailing list to alert people to upcoming sales. To get on it, ask for the Special Procedures Staff at your local office.

There are also other bargains, thanks to the U.S. government. The Bureau of Land Management will let anyone cut down a Christmas tree in many western national forests for about $1. For information, contact the Division of Forestry, Bureau of Land Management, U.S. Department of the Interior, Room 5620, 18th and C Streets NW, Washington, DC 20240.

And if you're a pond owner who lives in the Southeast, the U.S. Fish and Wildlife Service will supply you with free fish. Contact the Regional Director, Department of the Interior, Richard B. Russell Federal Building, 75 Spring Street SW, Atlanta, GA 30303.

Another tax deduction

Not only can married couples or single parents get a tax credit for a day-care center or nursemaid for a child in order to work, they are also entitled to a tax credit of up to 30 percent of the expense of sending the youngster to summer camp. It doesn't matter if the camp is a sleep-away or day camp; it is considered a form of child care and can be claimed under the Child and Disabled Dependent Care Credit Program. The child must be under fifteen to qualify. Total taxpayer income must be under $10,000 to qualify for the full 30 percent. The credit (Form 2441) is taken when filing Form 1040 at income-tax time in April.

Baby eyes

A special eyechart-testing technique has been devised for infants—one based on the fact that babies love to look at stripes. The chart employs two disks of light, one blank, the other striped, projected onto a screen. The eye doctor watches as your baby focuses on the stripes, and gradually makes the stripes thinner and more difficult to tell from the blank disk, at which point the baby starts looking at the blank circle just as much as at the fading stripes. It's a simple, quick screening test that can be performed in ten or fifteen minutes to catch ailments such as amblyopia (decreased vision). It's now being recommended that babies with some evidence of a vision problem be checked with this test.

Endometriosis therapy

Danazol is a relatively new synthetic hormone that's been developed for the treatment of endometriosis. That ailment, you'll remember, appears most frequently in women over 30, who should have a pelvic examination if they're considering having a baby. The new drug, said to be effective in most cases, is marketed under the brand name Danocrine.

Tooth saver No. 2

As you may recall, the best way to save a tooth that's been knocked out is to rinse it in water and pop it back into its socket. If that's not possible—young children may find it difficult to keep the tooth in place until they can get to a dental office—then put the tooth in milk, which is relatively bacteria-free. Researchers at the University of Florida report that milk even improves the chances of reimplantation. But, whether you tuck it into the socket or plop it into a cup of milk, get to the dental office immediately so that the dentist can put a splint on the tooth and attach it to the surrounding teeth for support while it reimplants itself.

APPENDIX A
Food Storage Guidelines

The following are suggested time limits for the storage of foods, after which oxidation and the action of enzymes will affect the quality of a particular food—its nutrition, flavor, color, and texture. Wholesomeness is not affected as long as the food is stored at freezer temperature, because bacteria do not multiply under such conditions. However, when thawing prior to cooking or serving, do not allow a food or its outer portion to reach the 45°–125° range for any length of time, because the bacteria would multiply to the point of dangerous contamination.

Shelf Storage (Unopened packages at cool room temperature)

BABY FOODS
9 months
custards and puddings
strained prunes
12 months
canned formula
18 months
strained apple, apricot, peaches,
green beans, spinach, mixed
vegetables, beef, pork, veal, liver,
chicken
20 months
strained pears, peas
25 months
strained carrots

FRUITS, CANNED
12 months
fruit pie fillings
18 months
cherries, maraschino and sour
grape juice
24 months
cherries, sweet dark
cranberry sauce
30 months
cherries, sweet light
grapefruit
plums
33 months
apricots
fruit cocktail
pineapple
36 months
apples, applesauce, apple juice
orange juice

peaches
pineapple juice
40 months
pears

VEGETABLES, CANNED
18 months
tomato paste
sauerkraut
24 months
beets
olives, green or ripe
tomato juice
30 months
mushrooms
potatoes, sweet or white
tomatoes
33 months
spinach
36 months
asparagus
beans, green
beans with pork, tomato sauce
42 months
carrots
corn, cream or whole kernel
peas
48 months
beans, kidney

MEATS, FISH, CANNED
18 months
sardines
24 months
tuna (water pack)

259

30 months
tuna (oil pack)
salmon
36 months
chicken
luncheon meat
42 months
corned beef

CONDIMENTS
18 months
jam, jelly
mustard, prepared
24 months
catsup
pickles, cured, in jar
sauces: hot, meat, soy,
Worcestershire

STAPLES, CANNED, IN JARS OR DRY
2 weeks
potato chips, package
3 months
popcorn, cellophane bag
6 months
mayonnaise
mixes for baked goods
olive oil (can)
12 months
baking powder
cereal, quick-cooking or dry

coffee, ground
cooking oil (can)
flour, wheat and rye
gelatine, flavored
milk, evaporated
pudding mixes, regular and
instant
18 months
molasses
rice, instant, carton
sugar, brown and confectioner's
tea
24 months
cocoa powder, can
noodles
rice, regular, bag
shortening
syrup
30 months
vinegar
36 months
chili, can
coffee, instant
cornstarch
macaroni, spaghetti
peanut butter
soup, condensed, can
Indefinitely
baking soda, carton
food coloring
salt, regular
sugar, granulated

Refrigerator (about 40°; times given in days)

MEATS
bacon, sliced, 7–21
beef
   roasts, steaks, 3–5
   ground beef, stew meat, 2
cold cuts 3–5
fish, 1–2
franks, flexible pack, 21–35
hams
   boneless cooked, 7–14
   canned, 180–270
   smoked, 28
lamb roasts, steaks, 5–7
pork roasts, steaks, 3–5
poultry, 5
veal roasts, steaks, 3–5

DAIRY CASE PRODUCTS
butter, 30
cheeses (surface sealed)
   blue, 135
   cheddar, natural, 1 year
   cottage, 14
   processed, unsliced, 240;
   sliced, 180
   Swiss, natural, 360
cream
   half-and-half, 7
   pasteurized, 21–25
   sour, 14
   table, 10
   whipping, 10
eggs, 120

margarine, 60
milk, whole, 7
yogurt, 7

FRUIT
apples, 2–7 months
apricots, 7–14
bananas, ripe, 2–4
berries
    blueberries, 14–21
    cranberries, 30–90
    strawberries, 5–7
cherries, sweet, 10–14
grapefruit, 28
grapes, 21–28
lemons, 30–120
melons
    cantaloupe, 15
    watermelon, 14–21
nectarines, 14
orange juice, 7
oranges
    California, 35–56
    Florida, 60–90
    Temple, 10
peaches, 7–10
pears
    Bartlett, 7–14
    Bosc, Comice, 2–3 months
plums, 7–14
tangerines, 7–14

VEGETABLES
asparagus, 2–4
beans, green or wax, 2–4
beets, topped, 7–14
broccoli, 2–4
Brussels sprouts, 2–4
cabbage
    red and summer, 7–14
    winter, 30–90

carrots, mature, topped, 120–50
cauliflower, 7–14
celery
    northern-grown, 30
    California or Florida, 7–14
corn, chilled in market, 4–8
cucumbers, 3–7
garlic, 180–240
lettuce, wrapped, 14–21
onions
    Bermuda, 42–56
    globe, 180–240
    green, 3–7
    Spanish, 30–60
parsley, 7–10
peas, unshelled, 2–3
pepper, green, 8–10
potatoes, several months
radishes
    spring, topped, poly bag, 7–14
    winter, topped, 30
spinach, 2–4
squash
    fall and winter, 120–80
    summer, 7–10
sweet potatoes, 120–80
tomatoes, 8–12
turnips, 7–14

BAKED GOODS, ETC.
cookie dough, packaged, 90
pies, fruit, 3
rolls, brown-and-serve, 21
shortening, 5 years
syrup, 1 year
yeast
    active dry, 6 months
    compressed, 7 days

Freezer Storage (0°)

FRUITS AND VEGETABLES
8 months
asparagus, beans, cauliflower,
corn, peas, spinach
12 months
fruits: cherries, peaches,
raspberries, strawberries
fruit juice concentrates: apple,
grape, orange

MEAT
2 months
pork, cured; pork sausage
4 months
hamburger
ground lamb
pork chops
8 months
pork roasts

9 months
lamb roasts
veal cutlets, chops
veal roasts
12 months
beef roasts, steaks

POULTRY
3 months
chicken livers
6 months
duck, whole
turkey, cut up
9 months
chicken, cut up
12 months
chicken, whole
turkey, whole

FISH
3 months
ocean perch fillets
sea trout, striped bass, dressed
6 months
fillets: cod, flounder, haddock, halibut
12 months
shrimp

FROZEN DESSERTS
1 month
ice cream, sherbet

APPENDIX B
Food-Drug Interactions

Drug (generic name)	Some common examples	Foods that may react with the drug
acetaminophen	Datril, Nebs, Tempra, Tylenol, Valadol	jelly, dates, crackers and other carbohydrates
bisacodyl	Bisal, Biscolax, Delco-lax, Dulcolax	milk and milk products
chlorpropamide	Diabinese	alcoholic beverages
demeclocycline	Declomycin	milk, dairy products, foods high in iron
digoxin	Lanoxin, Lauxin, Vanoxin	high-fiber foods such as bran; prune juice
erythromycin	E-Mycin, Ilotycin, Robimycin	acidic fruit juices, wines, syrups
griseofulvin	Fulvicin-U/F, Grifulvin V, Grisactin, Gris-PEG	foods high in fat, such as bacon, pork, butter, and margarine
iron (ferrous sulfate or ferrous chloride)	Feosol, Fergon, Iberet	milk, eggs, cereals, dairy products
levodopa (L-Dopa)	Dopar, Lavodopa	foods high in pyridoxine: dry skim milk, beans, oatmeal, wheat germ, beef liver, pork, tuna, sweet potatoes, peas, avocado, bacon, malted milk, salmon, walnuts
lincomycin	Lincocin	do not take with any foods (may cause diarrhea)
lithium	Eskalith, Lithane, Lithionate, Pfi-Lith	caffeine
lorazepam	Ativan	caffeine
methenamine mandelate	Mandelamine	citrus fruit juices, almonds, buttermilk, chestnuts, coconut, cream, fruit (except cranberries, plums, and prunes), milk

Drug (generic name)	Some common examples	Foods that may react with the drug
metronidazole	Flagyl	alcoholic beverages
Monoamine oxidase (MAO) inhibitors (furazolidone, iproniazid, isocarboxazid, mebanazine, nialamide, pargyline, phenelzine, pheniprazine, phenoxypropazine, piohydrazine, tranylcypromine)	Furoxone, Marplan, Niamid, Eutonyl, Nardil, Parnate Actomol, Catron, Drazine, Marsilid, Tersavid	foods high in tyramine: cheddar, Stilton, and Gruyère cheese, chicken liver, beer, wine, chocolate, avocado, soy sauce, raisins, pickled herring
penicillin		acidic beverages, such as citrus fruit juices, soft drinks, wine; aged cheeses
phenytoin	Dilantin, Diphentoin, Diphenylan, Toin	monosodium glutamate (MSG)
quinidine	Quinidate, Quinidex, Quinaglut	Same as for methenamine mandelate
tetracycline	Achromycin V, Cyclopar 500, Panmycin, Robitet, Sumycin, Tetracyn, Achromycin, Amtet, Bicycline, Bristacycline	Same as for demeclocycline
theophylline (aminophylline, oxtriphylline)	Amesec, Amodrine, Bronkaid, Bronkotabs, Kiophyllin, Quibron	caffeine
thyroid preparations	Armour Thyroid, Proloid, S-P-T, Thyrar, Thyrobrom	avoid long-term use of soy-protein products and cabbage, kale, Brussels sprouts, cauliflower, carrots, spinach, pears, peaches, and turnips
tolazamide	Tolinase	alcoholic beverages
tolbutamide	Orinase	alcoholic beverages

Drug (generic name)	Some common examples	Foods that may react with the drug
warfarin	Coumadin, Panwarfin, Athrombin-K	foods high in vitamin K, such as spinach, cabbage, cauliflower, kale, Brussels sprouts, potatoes, citrus, fish, liver

APPENDIX C
50 Common Harmful Plants

Cultivated house and garden plants	Toxic parts	Symptoms produced
1. **Caladium** *Fancy-leaf caladium*	All parts (toxic substance: calcium oxalate crystals)	Intense irritation to mucous membranes, producing swelling of tongue, lips, and palate
2. **Colocasia** *Elephant ear, Dasheen*	Same as above	Same as above
3. **Dieffenbachia** *Dumb cane, Elephant ear*	Same as above	Same as above
4. **Monstera** *Swiss-cheese plant, Ceriman*	Same as above	Same as above
5. **Philodendron** *Elephant ear*	Same as above	Same as above
6. **Ricinus communis** *Castor bean, Castor-oil plant, Palma Christi*	Seed, if chewed (toxic substance: ricin)	Burning sensation in the mouth, nausea, vomiting, abdominal pain, thirst, blurred vision, dizziness, convulsions
7. **Lantana** *Lantana*	All parts, especially the green berries (toxic substance: lantadene A)	Vomiting, diarrhea, weakness, ataxia, visual disturbances, and lethargy
8. **Lantana** *Hens-and-Chicks*	Same as above	Same as above
9. **Lantana** *Bunchberry*	Same as above	Same as above
10. **Hedera helix** *English ivy*	All parts (toxic substance: hederagenin, or steroidal saponin)	Local irritation, excess salivation, nausea, vomiting, thirst, severe diarrhea, abdominal pain

Cultivated house and garden plants	Toxic parts	Symptoms produced
11. **Digitalis** *Foxglove*	Leaves, seeds, flowers (toxic substances: cardioactive glycosides— digitoxin, digoxin, gitoxin, and others)	Local irritation of mouth and stomach, vomiting, abdominal pain, diarrhea, cardiac disturbances
12. **Rhododendron** *Rhododendron*	All parts (toxic substance: andromedotoxin)	Watering of eyes and mouth, nasal discharge, loss of appetite, nausea, vomiting, abdominal pain, paralysis of the limbs, and convulsions
13. **Rhododendron** *Azelea*	Same as above	Same as above
14. **Delphinium** *Larkspur, Crowfoot*	All parts, especially the seeds (toxic substance: delphinine)	Burning and inflammation of mouth, lips and tongue, followed by numbness; paresthesia, beginning in the extremities, progressing to entire body
15. **Delphinium**	Same as above	Same as above
16. **Hydrangea macrophylia** *Hydrangea*	Leaves and buds (toxic substance: Cyanogenic glycoside—hydragin)	Nausea, vomiting, abdominal pain, diarrhea, difficulty breathing, muscular weakness, dizziness, stupor, and convulsions
17. **Pyrus sylvestris** *Apple*	Seeds (toxic substance: cyanogenic glycoside—hydrangin)	Nausea, vomiting, abdominal pain, diarrhea, difficulty breathing, muscular weakness, dizziness, stupor, and convulsions
18. **Convallaria majalis** *Lily of the valley*	All parts (toxic substance: cardioactive glycoside—convallamarogenin)	Local irritation of the mouth and stomach, followed by vomiting, abdominal pain, diarrhea, persistent headache and cardiac disturbances
19. **Lathyrus odoratus** *Sweet pea*	Pea or seed (toxic substance: beta-[gamma-L-glutamyl]-amino-propionitrile)	Slowed and weakened pulse, depressed and weakened respiration, and convulsions

Cultivated house and garden plants	Toxic parts	Symptoms produced
20. Ipomoea violaces *Morning glory*	Seeds (toxic substances: several alkaloids that are chemically related to lysergic acid diethylamide, or LSD)	Hallucination-like states, nausea, loss of appetite, abdominal pain, explosive diarrhea, frequent urination, and depressed reflexes
21. Hyacinthus orientalis *Hyacinth*	Bulb; leaves and flowers if eaten in large quantities (toxic substance: unidentified)	Nausea, vomiting, abdominal pain, and diarrhea
22. Ilex *Holly, Christmas holly* Ilex vomitoria *Yaupon holly*	Bright red berries (toxic substance: unidentified)	Nausea, vomiting, abdominal pain, and diarrhea
23. Iris *Iris*	Rootstalk or rhizome (toxic substance: unidentified)	Nausea, vomiting, abdominal pain, and diarrhea
24. Ligustrum *Common privet*	Leaves and berries (toxic substance: unidentified)	Nausea, vomiting, abdominal pain, and diarrhea
25. Ligustrum *Waxed-leaf ligustrum*	Same as above	Same as above
26. Narcissus *Narcissus*	Bulb (toxic substance: unidentified)	Nausea, vomiting, abdominal pain, and diarrhea
27. Narcissus *Daffodil*	Same as above	Same as above
28. Narcissus *Jonquil*	Same as above	Same as above
29. Poinciana gilliesil *Poinciana, Bird-of-Paradise*	Green seed pods (toxic substance: unidentified)	Nausea, vomiting, abdominal pain, and diarrhea

Cultivated house and garden plants	Toxic parts	Symptoms produced
30. Wisteria *Wisteria*	Whole pods or seeds (toxic substances: resin and glycoside wisterin)	Nausea, vomiting, abdominal pain, and diarrhea
31. Nerum oleander *Oleander*	Leaves, stems and flowers (toxic substances: cardioactive glycosides—oleandroside, oleandrin, and nerioside)	Local irritation to mouth and stomach, vomiting, abdominal pain, diarrhea, and cardiac disturbances
32. Taxus *Japanese yew*	Seeds and leaves (toxic substance: alkaloid toxine)	Gastroenteritis and cardiac disturbances
33. Prunus americana *American plum, Wild plum*	Leaves, stems, bark and seed pits (toxic substances: cyanogenic glycosides)	Nausea, vomiting, abdominal pain, diarrhea, difficulty in breathing, muscular weakness, dizziness, stupor, and convulsions
34. Prunus armeniaca *Apricot*	Leaves, stem, bark and seed pits (toxic substances; cyanogenic glycosides)	Nausea, vomiting, abdominal pain, diarrhea, difficulty in breathing, muscular weakness, dizziness, stupor, and convulsions
35. Prunus virginiana *Choke cherry*	Leaves, stems, bark, and seed pits (toxic substances: cyanogenic glycosides)	Nausea, vomiting, abdominal pain, diarrhea, difficulty in breathing, muscular weakness, stupor, and convulsions
36. Solanum pseudocapsicum *Jerusalem cherry, Natal cherry*	All parts (toxic substances: leaves contain cardioactive substance solanocapsine; berries contain glycoalkaloid solanine and related glycoalkaloids)	Cardiac depression
37. Daphne mezereum *Daphne*	All parts, especially berries, bark and leaves (toxic substance: daphnin)	Local irritation to mouth and stomach, nausea, vomiting, and diarrhea
38. Rheum raponticum *Rhubarb*	Leaf blade (toxic substance: oxalic acid)	Corrosive action on the gastrointestinal tract

Cultivated house and garden plants	Toxic parts	Symptoms produced
39. Arisaema triphyllum *Jack-in-the-Pulpit, Indian turnip*	Leaves (toxic substance: calcium oxalate crystals	Corrosive action to gastrointestinal tract, producing swelling of tongue, lips, and palate
40. Podophyllum peltatum *Mayapple, Mandrake, Ground lemon*	Rootstalk, leaves, stems, and green fruit (toxic substance: podophyllo- resin)	Abdominal pain, vomiting, diarrhea, and pulse irregularites
41. Cicuta maculata *Water hemlock, Spotted cowbane, Poison parsnip*	Root and rootstalk (toxic substance: cicutoxin)	Increased salivation, abdominal pain, nausea, vomiting, tremors, muscle spasms, and convulsions
42. Parthenocissus quinquefolia *Virginia creeper, American ivy*	Berries and leaves (toxic substance: oxalic acid)	Corrosive action to gastrointestinal tract, nausea, vomiting, abdominal pain, diarrhea, and headache
43. Conium maculatum *Poison hemlock, Fool's parsley, False parsley*	All parts (toxic substances: lambda- coniceine, coniine, n-methyl coniine)	Gastrointestinal distress, muscular weakness, convulsions, and respiratory distress
44. Datura meteloides *Moonflower, Angel's trumpet, Locoweed*	Leaves, flowers, nectar, seeds (toxic substances: belladonna alkaloids)	Dilated pupils, dry mouth, increased body temperature, intense thirst, confusion, delirium, hallucinations, and pulse disturbances
45. Datura stramonium *Jimsonweed, Jamestown weed, Thorn apple, Angel's trumpet*	Same as above	Same as above

Cultivated house and garden plants	Toxic parts	Symptoms produced
46. **Robinia pseudoacacia** *Black locust, White locust*	Young leaves, inner bark, seeds (toxic substances: robin and robitin)	Nausea, vomiting, and abdominal pain
47. **Phytolacca americana** *Pokeweed, Pokeroot, Poke salad, Inkberry*	All parts, especially the root, leaves, and green berries (toxic substance: tannin)	Oral burning sensation, sore throat, nausea, vomiting, and blurred vision
48. **Gelsemium sempervirens** *Yellow jessamine, Carolina jessamine*	All parts (toxic substances: alkaloids—gelsemine, gelsemicine)	Cardiac depression, visual disturbances, dizziness, headache, and dryness of mouth
49. **Solanum dulcamara** *European bittersweet, Climbing nightshade*	Leaves and berries (toxic substance: solanine)	Vomiting, diarrhea, abdominal pain, drowsiness, tremors, weakness, and difficulty in breathing
50. **Atropa belladonna** *Deadly nightshade*	All parts (toxic substances: tropane alkaloids, atropine, and hyoscyamina)	Fever, visual disturbances, burning of mouth, thirst, dry skin, headache, and confusion

Permission to reprint this chart granted by the National Poison Control Network, Children's Hospital of Pittsburgh

APPENDIX D
Drug-Nutrient-Food Chart

Drug	Nutrient affected	Food to compensate
alcohol	folic acid	yeast
	vitamin B$_6$	wheat germ, meat, liver, whole grains, peanuts, corn
	zinc	oysters, liver, wheat germ, yeast, seafood
	magnesium	whole grains, legumes, water
antacids (containing aluminum hydroxide)	phosphorus	liver, eggs, milk, nuts
anticoagulants	vitamin K	leafy green vegetables
anticonvulsants	vitamin D	fish liver oils, fortified milk, butter, liver, sardines
	folic acid	yeast
aspirin	iron	liver, oysters, green leafy vegetables, dried apricots, prunes, whole grains, nuts
	folic acid	yeast
birth control pill	vitamin C	citrus fruits, rose hips, green peppers
cholestyramine (cholesterol-lowering medication)	vitamin A	liver, butter, egg yolks, deep yellow and orange fruits
	vitamin E	wheat germ, vegetable oils
	vitamin K	alfalfa
cigarettes (nicotine)	vitamin C	citrus fruits, strawberries, tomatoes, broccoli, cabbage
	vitamin B$_6$	liver, whole grains, soybeans, corn
	vitamin B$_{12}$	organ meats, fish, pork, eggs, cheese, milk and milk products

Drug	Nutrient affected	Food to compensate
corticosteroids	vitamin D	fish liver oil, fortified milk, liver, sardines
	vitamin B_6	wheat germ, meat, liver, whole grains, peanuts, soybeans, corn
	zinc	oysters, liver, wheat germ, yeast

Reprinted by permission of the *Nutrition and Health* newsletter of the Institute of Human Nutrition, Columbia University.

FYI PRODUCTION STAFF

Producer	YANNA KROYT BRANDT
Coordinating Producer/Writer	MARY ANN DONAHUE
Director	MICHAEL GARGIULO
Head Writer	LINDA KLINE
Director of Research/ Writer	JOE GUSTAITIS
Researchers/Writers	ELAINE BROWN WHITLEY, ROBIN WESTEN
Field Producers	ANDREW COMINS, JANE CHAPLINE, NEIL O'DONNELL
Photography Editor	NANCY BRENNER
Photographers	GIL ORTIZ, PETER CLEMENS
Business Manager	GREG MASON
Assistant Business Manager	DELPHINE SNIPES
Assistant Producer	SAL MANIACI
Assistant to the Producer	SHARON FISHER
Production Staff	JUDITH MARY GEE, JOHN PAUL WARD
Opening Title Sequence/ Creative Consultant (1980–1982)	ELINOR BUNIN

FYI CONSULTANTS

Child and Adolescent Psychiatry	DR. WILLIAM ELLIS. Child psychiatrist. Associate Professor of Child Psychiatry, Columbia University—Harlem Hospital affiliate.
Dentistry	DR. STEPHEN J. MOSS. Practitioner in pediatric dentistry, New York City. Professor and Chairman, Department of Pedodontics, New York University Dental Center. Past President, American Academy of Pedodontics.
Economics	REVA CALESKY. Financial counselor/accountant, tax specialist. Frequent lecturer on business and personal financial management.
General Medicine	DR. H. JACK GEIGER. Arthur C. Logan Professor of Medicine, City College of New York.

Director, Program in Health, Medicine and Society, School of Bio-Medical Education, City College of New York.

Nutrition

RUTH LOWENBERG. Program Development and Training/Supervisor, Nutrition Education Specialist, Cornell University, Cooperative Extension. Registered dietitian and Master of Science, Nutrition.

Obstetrics and Gynecology

DR. SHELDON H. CHERRY. Associate Clinical Professor of Obstetrics and Gynecology, Mount Sinai School of Medicine. Author of *Pregnancy and Childbirth* and *For Women of All Ages.*

Ophthalmology

DR. ROBERT WARD KLEIN. Director of Ophthalmology, Goldwater Memorial Hospital. Clinical Instructor, Ophthalmology, New York University School of Medicine.

Pathology and Laboratory Medicine

DR. RAYMOND GAMBINO. Director of Laboratories and Chief Pathologist, St. Luke's–Roosevelt Hospital Center. Editor, *Lab Report for Physicians.*

Pediatrics

DR. RAMON MURPHY. Assistant Professor, Clinical Pediatrics, Mt. Sinai School of Medicine. Director, Pediatric Poison Control Program. Fellow of the American Academy of Pediatrics.

Psychology

DR. MAGDA DENES. Clinical Professor, Adelphi University and New York University Faculty, and Supervisor, Mt. Sinai School of Medicine, Department of Psychiatry. Author of *In Necessity and Sorrow: Life and Death in an Abortion Hospital.*

PEGGY PAPP. Family therapist, marriage counselor, Ackerman Institute.

Sexual Help

LORNA SARREL. Assistant Clinical Professor of Social Work in Psychiatry, Yale University School of Medicine. Contributing editor to *Redbook* magazine.

DR. PHILIP SARREL. Associate Professor of Obstetrics and Gynecology and Psychiatry, Yale University School of Medicine. Contributing editor to *Redbook* magazine.

About the Editor

Nat Brandt's extensive career as a journalist has included work in radio and television and for newspapers, magazines, and a book company. He was a writer for CBS News in New York before entering the newspaper field, first as a reporter on several newspapers in Connecticut and New Jersey, then as an editor on the National News Desk of *The New York Times*. He subsequently was the managing editor of *American Heritage* magazine and the editor-in-chief of *Publishers Weekly*.

Mr. Brandt has edited books by, among others, William Saroyan and S. L. A. Marshall. Photographs from his travels around the world have appeared in *Life International, Horizon,* and numerous books and encyclopedias. His articles have appeared in *American Heritage, The New York Times Sunday Magazine, Redbook, Reader's Digest,* and other publications.

In addition to his current freelance activities, Mr. Brandt is an adjunct professor of communications at St. John's University in New York, where he teaches journalism and lectures on the mass media.

Index

Rathje, William, 78
Reading, 85, 217-218
Relaxation, 254-255
  and acne, 9
Remarriage, 151-152
Respite care, 16
Retinopathy, 44
Retired Senior Volunteer Program, 162
Retirement planning, 197-198
Reye's Syndrome, 44-45
Rheingold, Harriet L., 245
Rhythm method, 219-220
Riessman, Frank, 240
Ritodrine, 22
Rocking (babies), 49
Roller skating, 128-129
Rooney, Mickey, 179
Rosenberg, Elinor, 151
Rosenman, Ray H., 144
Rotter, Julian B., 98-99
Rubin, Lilian B., 101

Safety equipment, 60-61
Sager, Clifford, 152
Salt
  baby food, 50
  and colds, 222-223
  and hypertension, 13
  and moods, 20
Sanders, Shirley, 190-191
SATs, 75-76
Schachter, E. Neil, 248-249
School districts, 195-196
School lunches, 80-81
Schroeder, Carolyn, 154
Sciatica, 106
Scott, Alan B., 93-94
Scurvy, 106-107
Seat belts, 218-219
Second Opinion Hotline, 59
Security blankets, 187-188
Seelig, Mildred, 181
Self-care groups, 240
Self-help groups, 240-241
Sells, Lucy, 62
Serotonin, 19-20
Sexual drive, 147-148
Sexual vocabulary
  and children, 136-137
Shared-housing, 73-74
Shatin, Leo, 70-71
Sheehan, David V., 237
Shoes, 106
Showering (couples together), 213-214
Shyness, overcoming, 164-165
Sickle cell anemia, 147, 192-193

Sinanan, Kenneth, 77
Singing (to infants), 48-49
Sinusitis, 249
Skin moisturizers, 228-229
Sleeping pills, 254
Slipped-disk, 91-92
Small, Arnold, 213
Smoking, 165-166
  and hypertension, 13
Sneakers, 60-61
Sollie, Donna L., 66
Spider mites, 167
Spira, Melvin, 167-168
Sports-related injuries, 60-61
Spyker, Daniel, 242
Steam vaporizers, 235
Steinberg, William M., 251
Stepparents, 152
Sterilization, reversal, 113-114
Strep throat, 254
Stress
  and memory, 145
  and migraines, 40
Strokes, 130-131
Sugar
  and bacterial infections, 37-38
  and moods, 20
Suicide, 137
Sunglasses, 103-104
Sunscreens, 228-229
Surgery
  elderly, 33-34
  fetal, 22-23
  laser, 43-44
  plastic, 167-168
Sutton, J. R., 86
Swayback, 56
Swearing (children), 128
Swimming, 214-215

Tactile Communicator, 14
Talcum powder, 97-98
Talking
  to babies, 84-85
  to oneself, 190-191
Tarkenton, Fran, 85
Tax credit (summer camp), 257
Tearing (eyes), 123-124
Television watching, 114-115
TEL-MED, 58-59
Temper tantrums, 170-171
Tempo (music), 71
Testicular cancer, 112-113
Testosterone levels, 86, 148, 180-181
Thurston, Jean Holowach, 51-52
Thyroid, 9-10, 29

283

MP11N